Macrobiotics
for All Seasons

Macrobiotics for All Seasons

Vegan Recipes for Year-Round Health and Happiness

Marlene Watson-Tara

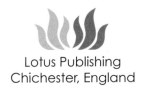

Lotus Publishing
Chichester, England

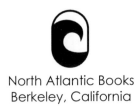

North Atlantic Books
Berkeley, California

First published in 2012. This edition published in 2013 by
Lotus Publishing
Apple Tree Cottage, Inlands Road, Nutbourne, Chichester, PO18 8RJ and
North Atlantic Books
P O Box 12327
Berkeley, California 94712

Photographs Marlene Watson-Tara
Text Design Wendy Craig
Cover Design Paula Morrison
Printed and Bound in the UK by Scotprint

Macrobiotics for All Seasons: Vegan Recipes for Year-Round Health and Happiness is sponsored by the Society for the Study of Native Arts and Sciences, a nonprofit educational corporation whose goals are to develop an educational and cross-cultural perspective linking various scientific, social, and artistic fields; to nurture a holistic view of arts, sciences, humanities, and healing; and to publish and distribute literature on the relationship of mind, body, and nature.

British Library Cataloguing-in-Publication Data
A CIP record for this book is available from the British Library
ISBN 978 1 905367 35 1 (Lotus Publishing)
ISBN 978 1 58394 558 2 (North Atlantic Books)

Library of Congress Cataloging-in-Publication Data
Watson-Tara, Marlene, 1957-
Macrobiotics for all seasons : vegan recipes for year-round health and happiness / Marlene Watson-Tara.
 p. cm.
 Summary: "In *Macrobiotics for All Seasons*, the unique and modern approach to macrobiotic eating—which explores the philosophy of the five elements and Chinese medicine and explains the health benefits of eating a diet that changes with the seasons—is shared"— Provided by publisher.
 Includes bibliographical references and index.
 ISBN 978-1-58394-558-2
 1. Macrobiotic diet. 2. Macrobiotic diet—Recipes. 3. Vegetarian cooking. I. Title. II. Title: Vegan recipes for year-round health and happiness.
 RM235.W38 2013
 641.5′636—dc23
                              2012023072

Dedicated to Mum – alias "Wee Mary" – with much love and gratitude
You truly are a girl of all "seasons"

Contents

Foreword

As a teacher of the macrobiotic way to health, I have given seminars and provided health counseling all over Europe and in North America. Together with my wife, Eugenia, I have managed the Macrobiotic Institute of Portugal in Lisbon for more than twenty-five years.

It is with great pleasure and honor that I write the foreword for this new book from Marlene Watson-Tara, *Macrobiotics for All Seasons*. I am sure it will help a countless number of people achieve healthier and more loving and happier lives, through the application of natural/macrobiotic principles applied to diet and way of life.

I met Marlene many years ago in Lisbon. She was attending an international event I had organized with my old friend Bill Tara, Marlene's husband. I remember meeting her in the lobby of a hotel in Lisbon and was immediately impressed by her vibrant energy, genuine smile and elegant manners.

Over the last few years we have had the opportunity to share many different types of moments: she has taught at some of our international programs and we have travelled together. She and Bill have shared with me their vision of promoting a healthier society through their educational activities and writing.

Our friendship has grown stronger, and Marlene continues to impress me through her incredible stamina and drive, dedication, professionalism and compassion. She is a good example of what she conveys in her book – someone who certainly "walks the talk" of her life. This book will give you very valuable information about how to take care of yourself and about the planet we live on; furthermore, it contains over two hundred recipes as well as medicinal teas and home remedies for many different health conditions.

I realize that we are facing tremendous challenges of many kinds – biological, social and environmental, to name the most pressing. It is my deepest conviction that, if we are to cope with these difficulties, we need to think, live and eat in a totally different way. The recommendations put forward by Marlene are certainly in line with the latest research on health and environmental issues, as well as with a traditional view of life that acknowledges the deep connection between humanity and the environment that creates us all.

I sincerely hope that anyone reading these lines will now read and study this book and implement the recommendations in their life; it is very likely that they will change it forever.

Francisco Varatojo

Lisbon, 7th August, 2011

Acknowledgements

I am so grateful to all those who have gone before me and created such inspirational literature on Traditional Chinese Medicine and macrobiotics, which I continue to study.

To my friends and fellow teachers – Eugenia Varatojo in Lisbon, Christina Pirello in Philadelphia and Meredith McCarty in San Francisco – I express my appreciation for their wonderful cookbooks and informative workshops and lectures that guide us all towards good health. To Christina in particular, I would like to acknowledge the fact that, when I was writing my first book seven years ago and asked her if I could "borrow" some of her recipes, she said: "Sweetie, take and use whatever you need." Rather exceptional I would say. And to so many other amazing teachers out there who endow the world with access to information for us all to learn from – I acknowledge all of you.

Without the skills of the love of my life, Bill Tara, who – among his many talents – is the most incredible editor, this book would still be on my PC and five times the size! As well as being my husband, friend and love, he truly is the most incredible teacher of teachers but has always told me that I am "unteachable" so I have therefore studied with many other teachers instead! I guess it's a bit like trying to teach your children how to drive. We have a lot of fun working and teaching together and I wish to thank him for his huge contribution to the health of our world to which he has devoted more than forty-five years of his life, travelling the globe and educating thousands of people. He is my biggest inspiration.

I would like to acknowledge every single one of you who buy this book; you have the vision to see that the only way forward to achieving good health is to adopt a healthy attitude and lifestyle. Believe it can be done. When you believe something can be done, I mean *really* believe, your mind will find the ways to do it. Believing a solution exists paves the way to that solution.

I would like to thank my publisher, Jon Hutchings of Lotus Publishing, for giving me the opportunity to create this book, and my editor, Steve Brierley of Paragon Editing, for his careful insight and wonderful job in the editing.

Thank you and much appreciation to Amanda Cruise from Helensburgh, Frank Taylor from the Penninghame Foundation, Gerry Campbell, Glasgow and Clearspring in London for the beautiful photographs of my recipes. A huge thank you to Ray and Marie Butler from the Penninghame Foundation, Newton Stewart, Scotland for supporting my programs and workshops and for creating the beautiful cooking school with twelve hands-on cooking stations that allow all our students and clients to really enjoy and learn about food and how to cook it.

Last but not least, a huge thank you to my wonderful family – Mum, Jackie, Marguerite, Sandie, Shirley and Lainey – who let me try out my many recipes on them throughout the seasons. I love you all.

We should all acknowledge and thank our bodies each day for our continued good health and not take it for granted. Health is everything – without health, everything is nothing.

Introduction

Healing truly does start in the kitchen, and that is what inspired me to write this book. As many of you will agree, it is not always possible to have home-cooked natural food. We live in the "real world": we travel and we often have to eat what is available at the time. My husband, Bill, and I understand this since we travel frequently. Yet, we have no ailments, take no medicine, have great energy and maintain a very good level of activity. Energy and restful sleep will come naturally with great health when we look at how healing begins in the kitchen.

For some, it takes a short while to adjust to changing their diet, but gradually old paradigms melt away and a new, healthier and happier way of thinking develops instead. You will feel cleaner, more organized, happier and healthier than you ever could have imagined possible. Macrobiotics and Traditional Chinese Medicine (TCM) are like a never-ending journey. The more you learn, the more you realize how much you don't know. If you understand the importance of keeping your biological systems balanced – working properly in the most efficient way – your body can create a regenerating environment, instead of a *degenerating* environment.

As we look back upon our life we often realize that the moments in which we have truly lived are the moments when we have done things in the spirit of love. If we love what we do, it makes us happy, fulfilled and energized. Lucky me: I am blissed and blessed because I love my work. That work is to use my personal experience, observation and study to enrich people's lives by helping them improve their health. Much of that work is contained in the following pages.

As I was writing this book, I thought about all the people whose lives could be improved by simply using natural solutions to their ailments and those of their loved ones. Often it is the simple things that produce the best results – I see this weekly in my students and clients. The sad truth is that so many of us suffer poor health and unhappiness because we do not have simple and practical information on how to make positive and productive changes to our lives. Out of need springs desire, and out of desire springs the energy and the will to achieve this. I hope that this book can give you some ideas on how you can improve your health and maintain good health today and all year round. The happiest people don't have the best of everything: they *make* the best of everything.

Picture yourself experiencing a day on which all your physical, spiritual and emotional traffic lights are flashing green, and you feel alive with great energy, free of the usual aches and pains. What we eat is one of the primary factors in achieving that kind of life. This book is about taking responsibility for your health. It is uncomplicated and user-friendly … just like me.

> *If you don't take care of your body,*
>
> *where are you going to live?*

This thought-provoking question has been my mantra for many years: it is printed on the front of the apron I use in cooking classes. When we think about our bodies as our home from birth to death, our perceptions can change about how we treat them. Would you fill your house with junk? Would you never clean it up or wash the windows? Would you let it slowly fall apart around you and simply move from room to room? Probably not, but many of us treat our bodies with the same neglect. Most people take better care of their cars than their bodies.

What we eat says much about how we feel concerning life in general and ourselves in particular. This respect, or lack of respect, is reflected in our state of health. What we eat today is who we are tomorrow. When you start to think this way and regard your body as sacred and precious, then the will to cherish and nourish it will come easily. Highly processed food and junk food will become less appealing to you, because you will not wish to violate your body/home. The desire to keep your home clean and comfortable will become a habit.

Much of the information in this book is inspired by the macrobiotic way of life. This system of health care and personal development originated in Japan but is based on a traditional understanding of diet, health and well-being recommended by ancient peoples from all over the world. It is a modern interpretation that is not therapeutic but directed more to general daily use and health maintenance. One of the interesting things that I discovered is that the modern macrobiotic approach to eating is consistent with the conclusions of modern nutrition studies. The only difference is that the macrobiotic approach is not a rigid diet, but describes a different way of looking at food – a way that is simple to apply and takes into account the relationship between what we eat and the environment.

Human beings are part of the environment, not separate from it. Global warming and other environmental problems that we now face are a result of acting as if there was a separation. But this is not a new issue. For centuries human society has lost the sense of stewardship that many primitive peoples possessed; now is the time to renew that bond with nature. Eating well is one of the most impactful acts we can engage in to create a healthy planet. When we respect the life of every living creature, we discover what it means to be human. Regardless of our state of health, there are always things we can do to improve our body/home.

I was not blessed with children; however, it does not make me feel any less responsible for leaving a lighter footprint on the planet than if I had seven children, and for doing the best I can do while I am here. This is what motivates me and drives me forward with my vision for a healthy world. The greatest adventure you go on is to live the life of your dreams. You cannot always control what goes on outside, but you can always control what goes on inside by feeding your body with healthy, wholesome food.

The purpose of my work is to share information and clear up confusion for consumers. My consultations, classes and retreats are always focused on how to protect, improve and maintain good health for the individual and the family. It is my commitment to provide common sense and practical solutions that are in line with solid science. Health is too important to give it away to corporations and food companies.

I hope this book serves as a valuable resource for creating a diet that is healthy for you and the planet. But how can you hope to discover the new, without a spirit of adventure? Make this an exciting time, learning about new foods and how to cook them. It could be as simple as having one meat-free week per month; if thousands did this it would make a huge difference to the environment. Have fun.

In good health and with much love,

Marlene x

www.marlenewatsontara.com

Chapter 1

NOT ANOTHER DIET BOOK!

Most people who buy a book with either food or diet in the title have bought one before. Food is a hot topic. We are informed daily about foods that will prevent cancer or cause cancer, extend our lives or shorten them. Diet books are a sure winner. If I were smart I would call this book *Marlene's Quick-Fix Detox Plan*. There is a lot of information out there and most of it is confusing. A Google search on "food" brings up about six and a half million articles. Just as a frame of reference, that's almost one million more than a search on "sex." Who would have imagined that?

The overflow of information about food and diet has created a jumble of contradictions and advertising disguised as science. One of the things I hope to do in this book is to introduce you to some simple and practical ways to eat a healthy diet that satisfies the senses, is easy to understand and balances our personal health with the health of the planet. If we can do all that at the same time, why not try?

Food is fundamental – no food, no life. Adequate or inadequate supplies of food determine who lives and who dies. The same rule applies to the quality of food: low-quality food can ruin your health and shorten your life, and high-quality food promotes health and may even extend your life. We are lucky that we have a choice. While many of us are fortunate enough to not have to worry about where our next meal comes from, that question is foremost in the minds of millions. Looking at it from that perspective, food choice definitely has a moral and political edge.

Food, water and air are the primary resources for life. It is for this reason that what we eat has a powerful impact on every aspect of our being. Food production, manufacture and distribution affect individual and social health, the economy and the environment. Food is a basic need that is wrapped up in sensory desire, family and culture. Our choices of food may reflect our spiritual beliefs and even our version of history. Food is the mysterious root of many serious social problems, yet this fact is easily misunderstood by the most superficial concerns.

My Approach to Health and Healthy Eating

This book is all about how we can use simple and effective ways to improve our health. It isn't about a new fad diet or exercise regime but is based on wisdom that has been around for thousands of years. It is the approach that I have used for many years to help hundreds of people reclaim their health. This information has always seemed to me to be common sense, and after reading a few chapters I hope it will do so to you too. My approach is based on understanding the cycles of nature, the changing of the seasons and the rhythm of our daily life, and using that insight to create a healthier and happier way of being. It is also an approach to health and healthy eating that is environmentally sustainable, an aspect that is very important to me. (Note that for all the recipes in this book, the quantities of ingredients are given in the metric system as well as in the equivalent British Imperial system.)

As a child my passion for nature and animals gave me the greatest joy. The work I do has grown out of my affection for both. As a teenager I loved being active and was always interested in how I could stay healthy. I discovered at an early age that good nutrition and exercise were the most important keys. Even at the age of sixteen I incorporated kelp seaweed into my diet (much to the amusement of my friends) and would always be reading books on health at the local library.

This curiosity and study has deepened over the years. Over the past two decades I have devoted my working life to bringing to others awareness about what I have personally experienced and learned. These experiences have taught me what I passionately share with all my clients and students. Scientific research has proved time and time again that by changing our daily health habits we can not only improve our health but also avoid many of the illnesses that plague society. One of the most important areas of change involves the way we eat.

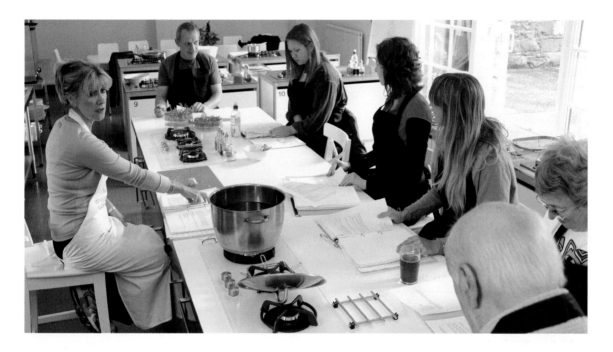

We all have immense resources for growth and change. I have seen many clients in their sixties and seventies change their dietary habits and find that debilitating ailments they have suffered with for years disappear. The old adage that "you cannot teach an old dog new trick" does not ring true.

My own mum, who is eighty-five years old, has the energy of someone in their sixties. If she has aches or pains or an upset stomach she calls me and I suggest simple "home remedies," and her ailments disappear. For someone suffering from chronic poor health, for which Western medicine offers no remedy, folk traditions often offer simple and effective alternatives. If we put ourselves back in charge and open ourselves to "alternative medicine" the outcome can be spectacular.

That is not to say that alternative or complementary medicine has all the answers. It is merely a fact that simple changes in personal health habits can have profound effects. Common illnesses – such as headaches, colds and flu, digestive upsets, and skin rashes – can be signals that our eating, drinking and lifestyle as a whole is "out of order." Instead of taking these messages on board and making the necessary adjustments, most people take medication to mask the symptoms. One of the many reasons why I love Eastern medicine is that when people learn the basics, they are learning skills for daily living that put them back in charge of their health.

Clients often say to me, "Why did I not meet you ten, twenty, thirty years ago? If I had known then what I know now my health would not be in the mess it is in today." I am devoted to helping people understand the simplest traditions of Eastern medicine in a way that is practical for modern living. This book, *Macrobiotics for All Seasons*, is a reflection of what I have found to be most practical and helpful. Over the years the positive outcomes of working with thousands of clients in this way have been so profound that I am motivated every day to share this work with as many people as possible.

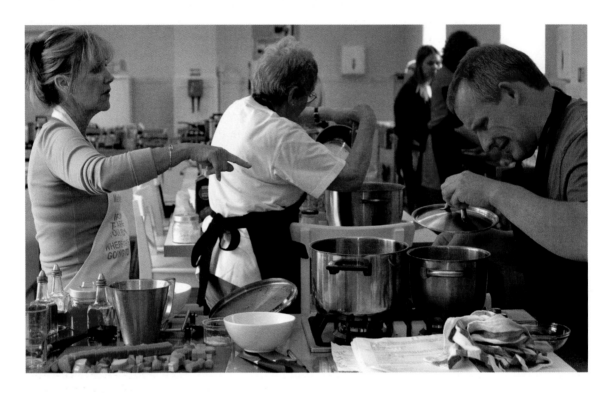

When clients tell me that they now have more energy, a healthy appetite, sound sleep, good memory and overall better health, it fills me with endless appreciation for the work I do and the understanding that what we teach works. Love and caring for family, friends and clients is what makes me "tick." They tell me it is like a new education, a new experience and a new life. The difficulties lie only in our social attitudes about health. When you challenge the status quo, many objections arise. It is almost as if you are offending people when you tell them that their health problems may be related to their diet. Modern thinking about disease is often based on fear and hostility, even as it becomes increasingly clear that cancer, heart disease and other chronic illnesses are more likely to be caused by personal lifestyle choices than by outside agents such as bacteria or viruses.

When I started my studies in Traditional Chinese Medicine, it was the biggest "Aha!" I had ever experienced – I took to the course like a duck to water. It was what I was meant to be doing with my life, from teaching chi ball, which is based on the Five Transformations philosophy, to teaching macrobiotic/natural foods cookery lessons, giving lectures and health consultations, and working with women's health – basically teaching people what I knew about Living with the Seasons. All of these activities are aimed at creating a balanced and healthy life. Living life to our fullest potential with great energy and vitality is what our body craves – it is how we are designed to be.

My approach to health is one that is firmly based on the relationship of the natural rhythms of the body to the planet we live on. We need this approach now more than ever since we seem to have lost touch with the lessons that nature has to teach us. No matter how much time we spend indoors, protected from the elements in our offices and homes, it is still our relationship with nature that rules our health. It is the natural world that is our home.

To be untouched by nature and the beauty of the seasons would, it seems to me, be like living our lives in a coma. To see cumulus clouds in a blue sky or watch the stars at night; a sunset, a sunrise, the moon shining on the water, the beauty of the mountains topped with snow ... so much to see, so much to be grateful for and all thanks to the seasons that bring us a landscape that never fails to please the eye. I always say thank you. One of my favorite pieces of music is Louis Armstrong singing "What a Wonderful World" – I know some people will think it's kitsch, but the words are beautiful and true.

Understanding our connection with nature can be difficult in today's world. We live in a culture that is fast paced and busy, busy, busy. It is often difficult to see the stars at night if we live in a city. Some years ago my brother-in-law John visited us in Portugal, where we were living and teaching. While we were sitting on the terrace he said, "God, look at the moon ... it is so beautiful. I can't remember when I last saw the moon." We have built a wall around ourselves, but nature is still there. The stars and the moon are still there even when we don't see them. The seasons rotate without much awareness on our part except a change in what we wear, but our body knows. Bringing this knowledge to the surface can help us build a better life.

Personal Health Care

Health is about freedom. Good health gives us the freedom to enjoy life more fully, to live the truth of who we really are. Here is a thought-provoking question I have asked many times: "If you don't take care of your body, where are you going to live?" Much of what holds us back is nothing more than habit. We get used to the way we live our lives and so does everyone around us. When we begin to make changes, it can rock the boat, and everyone gets nervous. The social pressure to be unhealthy is more overpowering than the encouragement to be healthy, which is why developing a healthy attitude is so important. But being healthy can be like swimming against the tide.

Try this. Tell your friends that you have decided to stop eating sugar or that you are going to start exercising daily, and see what happens. Make a mental note of how many people tell you that you'll never do it or that it can't make a difference. See how many of your friends are willing to share with you all the reasons why they have never done it, compared with those who are supportive.

It's just a matter of knowing what is really important to us and then making a plan to achieve it. Most of what gets in our way lies in the six inches between our ears. We are walking history books. All the information, attitudes and experiences of our lives are woven into a tapestry of habits, many of which don't make us healthy or happy. Making changes means taking a few of those strands and giving them a tug. If we don't like the pattern, we can change it. It's important to remember that we are not pretending to be doctors here; this is simply healthy living – treating sickness and living a healthy life are two different things.

> *The World Health Organization Definition of Health:*
>
> *"Health is a state of complete physical, mental and social well-being and not merely the absence of disease or infirmity."*

When we talk about health it invariably gets tangled up with the practice of medicine. I have no desire to be a doctor. In fact, the whole doctor-patient thing is a big part of the problem. We talk about health care and health services, but these are never about health – they are about sickness. The money that the government spends on health is really spent on sickness. Health care in America should be renamed the "Sickness Service."

Don't get me wrong, we need a sickness service – sometimes people need operations, drugs, MRIs and all of those wonderful modern techniques for dealing with serious illness or injury. We simply shouldn't confuse all of that with creating health. It's no use just muddling along till we get sick and then expecting the doctors to mend the damage. If we all wait until we get sick before we take action, we overload the doctors' surgeries, fill the hospitals, make our families and ourselves miserable and waste billions of dollars in the process. It's childish. We are all to blame. Why don't we just grow up and take care of ourselves? And we can, through one word: PREVENTION.

Here is a question for you. The bridge over a canyon collapses and cars are plunging into the abyss. There are two principal courses of action: (1) go down into the canyon and help those who are injured; or (2) stop the traffic first, then go down and help. It is a question of priorities. Our health service is in the canyon doing its best, but the cars keep coming, fast and furious. Someone has to stop the traffic. The solution is not going to come from the bureaucracy – they're down in the canyon counting the cars. The solution will come from creating a critical mass of individuals who are alert enough to look ahead, take responsibility for their health and put on the brakes. Some of those who stop will be brave enough to flag down the ones who are speeding by and get them to pull over too.

This health crisis exists because we are clamoring for more sickness service than can be logically provided. The pressure on the system creates a dangerous situation. In the National Health Service (NHS) of England and Wales, it has been reported that mistakes or "adverse events" in the delivery of health care are experienced in around 10% of inpatient admissions (Department of Health 2000, Vincent et al. 2001). It has been calculated that the human cost of these mistakes could be more than 40,000 lives a year, with a financial cost to the service of over £2 billion in additional care (Department of Health 2000). It was also widely acknowledged that there was significant under-reporting of deaths and serious incidents. An overtaxed system is a big part of the problem. It gets dangerous to be sick. This is not only a personal issue; it is reflected in the emotional and physical effect of disease on families and society. Each year sickness costs UK employers over £11 billion.

Look at the logic of this: heart disease and stroke are the top killers in the UK. They account for 39% of all deaths, followed by 26% for cancer and 13% for respiratory disease. This health crisis exists because we are clamoring for more sickness service than can be logically provided. The pressure on the system creates a dangerous situation. HealthGrades, a health care ratings company, has produced studies that show the huge impact of "medical error." Their research, published in the *Journal of the American Medical Association* in October of 2003, showed estimated deaths by error at 98,000 annually. Dr. Samantha Collier, vice-president of medical affairs, was quoted as saying: "The equivalent of 390 jumbo jets full of people are dying each year due to likely preventable, in-hospital medical errors, making this one of the leading killers in the U.S."

According to the Centers for Disease Control and Prevention, coronary heart disease alone was projected to cost the United States $108.9 billion. This total includes the cost of health care services, medications, and lost productivity. Remember that this is a largely preventable disease.

In fact cancer rates are still rising. My husband, Bill, and I attended a lunch recently where three out of four women there had lost their husbands to cancer – and at a young age! If the most conservative experts are correct, that means at least one of these men, more likely two, would still be alive if they had taken better care of themselves. This is also the case with diabetes.

The biggest health threat on the horizon is the increasing incidence of diabetes, a disease that is closely linked to rising rates of obesity. The problem is that the issue of obesity is often seen as a cosmetic issue, not a serious health problem. With obesity rates approaching 30% of the population in many areas, this is serious. This condition is linked not only to diabetes but also to heart disease and many cancers – it is also known to be directly connected to diet and exercise. These problems are largely preventable. That's right: they are diseases that we succumb to through the way we live. We regularly have clients for consultations who control their blood sugar, reduce cholesterol levels and establish a healthy body weight by following a simple program we design for them. It's so simple; it makes you wonder why this isn't followed in hospitals.

It is an unfortunate fact that most people wait until they are suffering before they take action. It's a pity, since the object of the exercise is to experience the joy of living life more fully. Living with the Seasons is simply about creating new habits that support the very best qualities of our life. These new habits can often make the old ones – the ones that hold us back – less appealing. Our habits did not simply fall out of the sky – we created them. The chocolate bar that undermines our weight loss is not hiding in the shop waiting to jump out at us – sometimes it may seem that way but, trust me, it isn't. The couch that gets selected over the brisk walk doesn't whisper sweet nothings in your ear – you choose it. So what do we do? We need to focus on creating a new way of life that has more long-term rewards by establishing a healthy rhythm to our life, one that reflects what our body needs. The rewards are huge.

Nutrition and the Macrobiotic Way of Eating

My interest in health and nutrition eventually led me to the macrobiotic approach to eating. When applied with common sense this is a very flexible way of eating. It reflects the connection between humanity and the planet – it is an ecological approach to eating and I love it.

Modern macrobiotic dietary principles have developed over the past fifty years in America, Europe and Asia. They are based on the philosophy of Asian medicine as practiced in China and Japan. These concepts reflect physical, environmental and social observations over a period of more than five thousand years. Although the philosophy bears little relationship to Western nutritional science, the conclusions are very similar.

While the diet most associated with macrobiotics is the "Standard Macrobiotic Diet," this method of eating is not a diet in the strict sense – it is a way of choosing foods for personal needs. Michio Kushi developed the standard diet in the early 1980s with assistance from my husband, Bill Tara, together with Ed Esko, William Spear and Murray Snyder (Kushi et al. 1981, available from the Kushi Institute).

The standard diet was developed to describe a general pattern of eating to the growing number of people seeking help with their health who were dealing with cancers, heart disease and a variety of serious illnesses. While thousands of people found assistance in recovering their health using variations on the standard diet, the association of macrobiotics and healing is often not clearly understood.

The application of macrobiotic principles to nutrition is not an attempt to therapeutically correct the symptoms of disease. The macrobiotic approach to eating focuses on assisting the body to recover from nutritional stress, often the result of the modern diet, and return to a more sensible state of biological balance. During the process of returning to a more balanced state, many people experience a natural recovery of health and in some cases a complete remission of serious symptoms. The diet helps the body exercise its own self-healing capacity. Some of the healing teas that may be used to accelerate that process are recommended in the following chapters. You will really enjoy using these teas – they are easy to make and very effective.

During the 1970s and 1980s, macrobiotic practitioners came under attack from some nutritionists, who criticized them as being "unscientific" and mistaken in their views that there was a direct connection between diet and serious disease. The focus of conventional nutrition on nutritional *deficiency* ignored the fact that the degenerative diseases of modern society are diseases of *excess*. The macrobiotic view has been proven true. The dietary recommendations that were generated by the macrobiotic community are reflected by those coming out of international bodies such as the World Health Organization Dietary Recommendations (WHO 2002) or by *The China Study* (a 2006 book by T. Colin Campbell, Jacob Gould Schurman Professor Emeritus of Nutritional Biochemistry at Cornell University, and his son, Thomas M. Campbell II). Men and women following the macrobiotic diet have been included in several studies carried out by Harvard Medical School (Sacks et al. 1975) and shown to display superior heart health to the general population. Now the tables have turned.

The overwhelming evidence of contemporary science is that food is a major contributing cause of many cancers, stroke, diabetes, heart disease and a variety of major illnesses. The particular dietary factor most implicated in this relationship is the overconsumption of meat, dairy products and simple sugars. Diets that are dominated by these foods are also usually devoid of whole-cereal grains, vegetable protein, adequate fresh vegetables and fruits, seeds and nuts.

The worldwide macrobiotic community has played an important role in advocating dietary reform, promoting organic farming, introducing Asian soy products and encouraging individuals and families to become more conscious of food choices and return to meals prepared in the home. This book is my contribution to that movement.

Chapter 2

HEALTHY HABITS

When you buy a new car there is an operation manual in the glove compartment. This is a good idea since cars are expensive and can easily be damaged if not cared for. The manual tells you what kind of petrol and oil to use, what to do when the warning lights come on, and how to change tires if you get a flat. It is unfortunate that we are not all issued with a similar manual when we are born, containing this kind of information for the human body. We just don't seem to know how to interpret those warning lights or what kind of maintenance plan to follow. It's like getting into a spaceship and being told, "It's all yours, take control – have fun." It is especially uncomfortable when we discover that the other passengers are just as clueless as we are.

The human body is a miracle in its design. It comes complete with thousands of self-healing and repair mechanisms. The key is finding out how to interpret the warning signals and how to maintain our health in the first place. If we don't have this information, we are apt to ignore important messages or feel we need professional advice every time we have a sniffle. That doesn't mean we don't require an expert on occasion. It simply means that we should all be able to manage our life in a healthy manner and avoid the avoidable.

Good health has been turned into a complex and mysterious thing, but it isn't. There are many actions we can take to improve our health and the only things that hold us back are habits, the fear of change and a lack of practical information. It's simple and straightforward (just like me). If we were given that operation manual at birth, it would have "Life Skills for Healthy Living" on the cover. I know a lot of what would be inside it. I know what I know because of what I've seen and experienced. We all deserve to be healthy and if we are willing to open our minds, we can achieve it. All that is necessary is desire and practical tools.

The diseases that most plague Western society are the degenerative diseases. The interesting thing about these problems is that they can often be prevented or managed by simple adjustments in daily living. It is the actions we take daily – our personal habits – that are the issue. Commenting on a recent report from the WHO (2011), Director-General Margaret Chan says that millions of people are dying prematurely every year from the world's biggest killers. These include cancers, heart disease, stroke, chronic respiratory disease and diabetes. The WHO reports that up to 80% of heart disease, stroke and type 2 diabetes, and more than one-third of cancers, could be prevented by eliminating the major risk factors.

We know what causes the most deaths. In a publication by the American Department of Health and Human Services in 1993, it was reported that two-thirds of premature deaths are caused by poor nutrition, physical inactivity and tobacco. That death rate is five times more than the number of people killed by guns, HIV and drug use combined. We also know that most common digestive disorders, obesity, insomnia, headaches and sexual dysfunction are caused by the same choices. We have to ask, why then are we not seeing these problems diminish? Part of the answer is simply that habits are hard to break.

Changing a Habit

What most of us do in the course of a day is habit. The way we brush our teeth, the way we pour our tea, the order that we put on our clothes are all habit. These small daily actions don't really cause us any problems, unless we decide to pull on our socks when our shoes are already on our feet, but in some areas of life, habits can have profound effects. As they say – the devil is in the details.

There are two major factors that inspire people to change their habits. Unfortunately the most common is fear. Once a diagnosis is made that our cholesterol levels are too high, our blood pressure has reached a dangerous level or our lungs are packing up, we may become motivated to change. This is good of course, but wouldn't it be more sensible to take positive steps before the ambulance arrives?

Another route to changing habits is to create a healthy vision of ourselves and make an action plan to achieve it. This means that we realize that our lives will be happier if we improve our health. What if we can be more active, increase our mental clarity or be more physically attractive? Wouldn't that be worth a little effort? I think so. Realizing the personal rewards of increased health is the best path.

It is interesting that when people are asked what it means to be healthy, they often use the word "balanced." The problem is that we don't often know what we are supposed to be in balance with. It is an important issue since health does have something to do with balance. It has to do with living a life where all aspects of our being fit together with the least amount of friction. We are not made up of independent and unrelated fragments. One origin of the word "health" means to be whole. Our body, mind and spirit do not exist in separate dimensions – the medical traditions of the Far East realized this. Life is seen as a series of relationships in which every aspect of being had an effect on everything else.

Imagine cutting an onion in half from the top to the bottom, with the layers of tissue exposed. Each of these layers is connected to the center. Our life is something like that. The environment, our culture, our family, our emotional and mental life and the functions of our physical self are all layers of one totality. What happens at any level of our growth and development affects all the rest. We all know this to be true. If you wake up in the morning with a head cold you may not be the same smiley person that usually walks into breakfast. You may feel like slamming the door or irritated by the time it takes for the kettle to boil. You may not be able to concentrate at work or may even feel depressed – all because of a blocked sinus. Let's take this simple example one step further.

What if your sinus is always blocked? What if you have simply become unaware of it as a problem and it has become "normal"? Does this mean that the feelings of irritation become normal too? This ought to be a warning light flashing and yet we keep on "driving." The results are never good. At best, the outcome is wear and tear, but repair, replacement or a breakdown could be on the horizon. It is the strain between our way of life and our basic human needs, coupled with our unconscious neglect of the warning lights, that makes up much of the tension we experience. We call this tension "stress."

Stress and the Challenge of Change

It often appears that we are suffering from a stress epidemic. Most of the clients we see for health counseling complain of suffering from stress. Their lives are filled with the pressures of family, work and community; they seem to have no time for themselves and have to push themselves to the limit. That is why many of them are looking for ways to increase stamina and simplify their daily routine. They realize that it is the joy we experience and the people we know and love that truly make this life journey colorful, rich and rewarding. They are facing the challenge of making changes and that's a big one.

Stress is one of the biggest health issues in modern life. It is a major factor in the development of many diseases and yet some people seem to be proud of being stressed out of their minds. After all, if you aren't stressed out you must be lazy. Even children talk about being "stressed out." We live in an age where the ability to multi-task and juggle a thousand things at once is a badge of courage. That pride wears thin when we start dropping the balls. What do we do then? Do we soldier on until we exhaust ourselves and get sick? Do we medicate ourselves so that we can keep up with the parade, sell everything and move to a cave, or do we learn to take charge of our lives and make the changes that will free us up?

We can reduce stress in our lives if we are willing to embrace change. What I have learned is that every change I have experienced is an opportunity to re-invent myself. Sometimes my changes have been overwhelming, but as I develop trust in myself and learn from the rhythms of nature, I find myself able to produce better outcomes – or at least to not get knocked off my feet. People, work, friends, living situations – anything can change. The good news is that we are not simply spectators or victims; we can make decisions, and we have the ability to choose. I like to say in the morning when I awake, "Today is a new day and I am a new me." I look forward to the day ahead and the new opportunities it offers.

I suggest that the best time to make changes in health habits is right now! It's not like we don't know what to do. In workshops we often ask people to write down the things they know they could change to be healthier – just a simple list of five to ten things. Guess what? Everyone can do it. You can do it right now in your head. Here are some golden oldies: lose weight, stop eating junk food, eat more fruit and vegetables, get more exercise, and spend more time relaxing with friends or family. All these things are easy if we show some commitment and have useful information on how to put them into practice. It is important that you don't make being healthy drive you crazy. Make it fun – this is an adventure and all you need is a map and a compass. You can use this book as a map, but your compass must be what *you* want to achieve. Establish your goal and stick with it.

Habits exist for a reason. They may be patterns of adaptation to the habits of those around us, ways of getting pleasure that we aren't getting anywhere else, or ways to comfort us or maybe even to escape. One thing is certain: the best way to change unproductive habits is to create new and better ones.

Accepting the challenge of change has a lot to do with establishing health. If you don't see that there are parts of your life that don't work and require attention, you cannot focus your energy towards fulfilling your true potential. Change requires some energy but is exciting and rewarding if we are truly committed. Change happens one step at a time. I did not change my health habits overnight; I experimented, studied and learned from people who were further along the road than I was.

The focus of this book is on the food we eat, but it would be silly to think that food is the only factor in leading a healthy life. Everything we do has an effect on our well-being. Let's look at some of the things that are important.

Create Goals and Identify the Benefits

Imagine that you knew your life was coming to an end but you were given the chance to live it all over again – what would you want to do more of? Would you want to work more, or spend more time watching TV or surfing the Internet? We often spend an inordinate amount of time doing things that add no real value to our lives. Sometimes it seems we are simply waiting till life is over as if this was a rehearsal. Life is no dress rehearsal and I always try to live each day as if it were my last, because one thing that is for sure – one day it *will* be.

There are areas of our lives that are essential and things that are not – where then do we invest our time and energy? Sleeping and working are the two activities that seem to take up most people's time. That might be all right if our work is fulfilling, but most people don't have fulfilling jobs. It is easy to waste time when we don't know what we want to do.

If we have a personal vision of our life the way we want it to be, then there should be some evidence that we really want it. How could we be better spending our time? My experience is that when people have a vision of their life that is meaningful, they find it easier to achieve health. The reason is simple – they want the vitality and well-being to make it happen. There has to be a benefit that has emotional impact. I have a sign up above my PC that I read every day. It says "Good morning, Marlene – there are unforeseen forces supporting your dreams." This makes me smile because I dream BIG, and for years and years my family has listened to me talking about what I want to create; these affirmations keep the energy alive around my vision.

Develop Health Allies and Nurture Positive Relationships

Making changes to our way of life has its challenges and we can all use all the help we can get. Keep on the lookout for people who are also interested in creating a healthy life, and form some partnerships. Go walking together; share health goals and support each other in your adventures. We can all learn from each other and it is good to know that you are not alone in your quest for a more healthy life.

Let your family and close friends know what you are doing and don't be critical of the fact that they are not ready to make the same changes as you. Many well-intentioned people become evangelists for healthy living right away and feel that they need to convert the world. Take care of yourself first and develop a sense of humor.

Dealing with other people's scepticism also needs to be addressed. If you are going to live a healthy life, be aware that others may not understand your actions. A good sense of humor and some humility are called for. Sharing food, drink and amusement are part of social bonding. If you start to refuse certain foods or drinks, it can be interpreted as an act of arrogance or judgement. It is your responsibility to keep it light. Being healthy doesn't mean you can't live in the real world; it also doesn't mean you should run blindly with the crowd. Everyone has their own decisions to make in their own time. Having said that, there will always be the friendly saboteurs.

The friendly saboteur most commonly comes in two varieties. The first is simply concerned for your well-being. When someone starts to try something new, there are questions. Is this safe? Are there hidden dangers? Is this some cult behavior? There will be concern that there is not enough protein in your diet, or that you might get scurvy or any number of imagined problems. The concern is genuine; there is simply an information deficit. This friendly saboteur simply needs information.

The second type of saboteur is perhaps more defensive than friendly. They may feel threatened by your decisions to change your routine. They are sometimes family members. They will tell you that what you are doing is nonsense, that it's dangerous, that it's antisocial. In fact, what they are doing is attempting to justify their own behavior. After all, if what you are doing is valid, what does that say about what they do?

I have had people tell me that I eat rabbit food, that my exercise regime is silly and that my affirmations are stupid. The fact that I never need to see a doctor or that my energy levels far exceed theirs and I am fifty-four years old doesn't seem to mean much; it does to me. I must be doing something right.

Keep Positive

Imagine the mind as the sum total of all you have experienced, learned and been told. These are all influences of the past – they may or may not be true for the present or the future. If we allow old experiences to dictate our actions, we become slaves to the past. This slavery holds us back from moving into a new future.

Ask yourself how often you were told that you couldn't accomplish certain things because you were too young, too old, a woman, a man, not smart enough, not good looking, and so forth. History is filled with men and women who rose above difficulty to accomplish great things. These people all had one thing in common: they didn't believe the dream-stealers and the negative folks around them. They also often failed many times before achieving success. These people are worth taking as models.

If we repeat a thought enough times, we start to believe it. Thoughts can become reality. If we are told something enough times, we begin to think it's true. If we fail at a task and are given a reasonable reason for our failure, we often embrace it. Whew! What's a poor girl to do? When we take in the myriad of excuses, rationales and unasked-for advice, we create a monkey mind.

The monkey mind is filled with thoughts that confuse, conflict with and contradict our intentions. We inherit some of the monkeys. Friends, parents and spouses – everyone is happy to share their favorite mischief-maker with you. I see the monkeys in operation every day in my own life and in the lives of others.

When someone comes to me for a health consultation, they fill out a form and we have a conversation about their health and their health goals. When we begin to talk about making changes, it is amazing how quickly the monkeys spring into action. I demonstrate a simple recipe for life change and out pops a monkey, "Oh, I can never do that."

They have never tried to do it before and yet, "Oh, I can never do that" pops right out. Of course they can do it. It is never difficult and with time they will succeed if they are motivated, but the struggle with the monkey will make it hard for them. Some people laugh and say, "Wow, that's interesting, I'll try." It is the more positive clients who get the best results. It's all about the monkeys.

Over the years we come to believe these monkey thoughts are true. When we build our world around them they of course become true. We need to recognize the monkey for what it is, and create some new programs to run with. The bad news is that we hardly ever lose those monkeys; the good news is that they don't need to run the show. We have the ability to create new images and beliefs if we want to.

Don't let other people undermine your quest for health; to be healthy is always going to mean going against the grain. The reason is simply because health is not common. Watch out for other people's monkeys and your own. Focus on what you want to accomplish and stick to it.

Create a Plan for Success

If you wanted to start a new business or plant a garden you would make a plan. You would decide what tools you needed and what you were going to do first, and then you would take action. It is interesting how many people never make a plan for the important project of creating better health.

You will probably never stop smoking if you keep buying cigarettes. If you want to eat only healthy food, why fill the kitchen with unhealthy food? Planning means making sure that your best intentions have a chance. If you know that there is a coffee break at work and people have a pastry and coffee, but you want to break that habit, why not bring a healthy snack? Make sure that you have tea or juice to drink – if not, guess what? The same is true with that carton of ice cream in the refrigerator – get rid of it. Plan your meals, learn to cook as soon as possible, and get up earlier or reduce the amount of TV viewing so that you have time to exercise.

If you follow the dietary and lifestyle suggestions in this book your health will improve. There is nothing that is difficult – the challenge is to take the practical steps to make it easier. Start by setting up a healthy kitchen, buying healthy ingredients, making menu plans and being creative with using leftovers to make it easy. Health is a big project and is worth the attention.

Get Daily Exercise

I have been a great fan of exercise all of my life, and some of my friends might use the word "fanatic" to describe me, but that's not true. I know that when you move your body, it rewards you with increased energy and flexibility. We have become a nation of couch potatoes. We watch over thirty hours of TV a week, but don't have the time to exercise. I'm not talking about getting your leg above your head or running three miles before breakfast. We all need to find the activity that suits our lifestyle, but we do need to find one.

Exercise is one of the best ways to reduce stress, improve cardiovascular condition, improve diabetes, and reduce bone loss in women and the elderly. This is not theory – it's a fact. We also know that children need plenty of exercise to keep their body weight down and to improve their general health. And our government's response to this? Cut down the number of opportunities for kids to engage in sport!

Most people get their maximum exercise from walking to the car or the bus from their front door – a distance they walk twice a day. When we are young it doesn't matter so much, but as we grow older it makes a huge difference. A small amount of daily exercise can mean the difference between a healthy life and a heart attack. It's important not to wait until it's too late.

This is not about "getting fabulous abs in ten days" or "losing twenty pounds in a week." It's all about being healthy, enjoying life, being able to play with the children or grandchildren and feeling enlivened instead of over the hill. It's not about looking like a model or a movie star – we have way too much of that. In fact, that's part of the problem.

Advertising and the media bury us with an avalanche of images showing us what is handsome, beautiful and desirable. It has lead us to a situation where women, and an increasing number of men, either try to starve and stuff themselves into a mold they never will fit, or simply give up and sink into the couch. This is not healthy. You can weigh more than you should and still be fit; you can lack perfectly sculpted muscles and still have vitality and flexibility.

It doesn't need to be complicated. Doing something like walking or riding a bike every day is more effective than going to a fancy gym once a week. Do things that you can fit into your life; doing something is better than doing nothing. Don't sabotage yourself. Did you know that most health clubs would go broke if people only paid when they used the facility? Most people buy a gym membership card, then don't bother to use it. Likewise, garages all over the world are filled with exercise equipment bought in a rush of enthusiasm and left to rust.

Eat Good Food

Since this book focuses on food, there is plenty in the following chapters about eating habits. The most important things are avoiding foods that are filled with chemical additives, focusing on locally grown foods where possible, trying to eat foods when they are in season and choosing plant over animal sources of protein. In the next chapter I will go into much more detail. Selecting healthy food is the single most important thing you can do to establish and maintain a healthy life.

Learn to Cook and Eat Slowly

Cooking is fast becoming a lost art. Oh, there are plenty of cooking shows on TV and there is no shortage of flashy cookbooks, but unfortunately they usually don't give you the information needed for following a healthy diet.

Cooking is the way that we process food in order to release the energy it contains. Through good cooking we can make food more digestible and tasty. We can preserve foods, improve their nutritional value, and combine them for better health.

Chewing and eating slowly are the perfect complement to good food choices and cooking. By cooking food, our ancestors externalized and extended the digestive process with conscious attention. Cooking allowed us to better digest and release the energy of the food we were consuming. When we chew our food well we enhance the digestive process as well. This is especially true if we are eating a wholefood diet. Modern processed foods often do not require chewing – they are manufactured purely for tasting and swallowing.

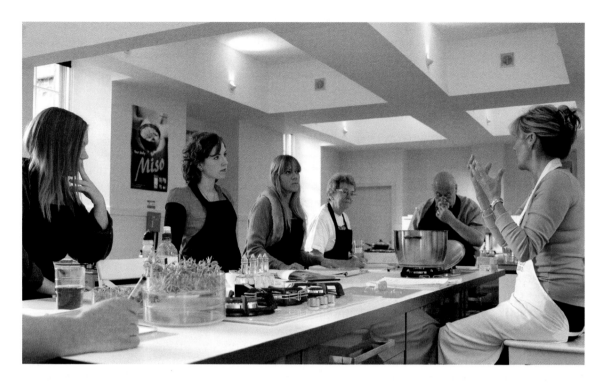

The modern habits of eating on the run, eating while standing and eating at irregular hours undermine the nutritional value of what we eat, cause digestive disruption and make us unaware of what we are eating. Good food, cooked well and eaten with respect, has the greatest health benefit.

Release Stress and Sleep Well

This seems to be just as much of a challenge as being active. Relaxation is not the same as falling exhausted into bed or slipping into a near-coma in the middle of a conversation. We seem to have lost the ability to simply let go and put the mind and body into neutral. If this is the result of our way of living, then we had better figure out how to get it under control or stop putting ourselves in this situation. It is well worthwhile to learn a simple form of meditation, stress release or visualization to assist relaxation.

Relaxation and deep, regenerative sleep are primary requirements for good health. During deep sleep we allow stress, held in the muscles of the body, to be released. It is the only time of the day when the immune system rebuilds. The lack of sleep is cumulative; getting one good night's sleep does not make up for one bad night. When we sleep, our mind alternates between deeper and shallower levels of sleep. With each repetition of this cycle our body becomes more and more relaxed. Disruptions to this cycle mean we never get the full benefit of sleep.

It is a well-known fact that poor sleep is a major cause of automotive accidents and work accidents; it is also a contributor to alcoholism. Often a person with a sleep problem begins drinking before bed. Over time the need for alcohol increases until a dependency is established; the same situation occurs with drugs.

What I know is that when we take charge of our life, eat well and get good exercise, the ability to relax during the day and sleep well at night is increased. This is particularly true when we use some of the folk remedy teas that I will be introducing in the following chapters; some of these teas will help you sleep better. Make sure that you don't watch disturbing programs or the news before going to bed. Try to get into the habit of reading something calming before sleep.

Unplug and Spend Time in Nature

We are increasingly becoming creatures who spend all their time indoors. It is essential that we make the time to get out of the house or office and go to the local park or take a trip to the country. Being in nature supports our appreciation of it and gives us the time and space to allow the environment to work its particular magic on us.

When we are in the forest or parkland, on the beach or near a running stream, the air is filled with negative ions. These charged particles actually support a positive attitude: they are vitamins for the brain. Fresh air, trees and flowers, sunshine and the sound of the breeze blowing through the leaves all nourish our being in a special way and contribute to our health. The opposite is true with much of the technology we are used to.

We are surrounded by technology and much of it requires our attention. It is easy to find ourselves constantly plugged in, and some of these electronic toys may be harmful to our health. There is a growing concern over the use of mobile phones because of the microwaves that they give off and the heat generated from their batteries. It is certainly true that young children should not use them too much, so why not show some caution and limit their use? Being in the moment is a healthy thing to do – unplug once in a while and you will feel better for it.

Chapter 3

THE MODERN DIET

Every chemical process in the body is dependent on our consumption of food, water and air. Since this is true, paying attention to what we eat is essential for good health. The problem is that eating well can be a challenge when shopping for food in the local supermarket. What we don't eat is just as important as what we do eat. I will give you lots of good ideas in the following chapters, but before that we have to take a look at some of the disaster zones in the modern diet. Let's get the bad news out of the way first.

Miracle cures, miracle foods and quick-fix diets flood the marketplace. Every few months a new diet hits the market. There are diets to improve your sex life, add muscle to a flabby body, flush the evil toxins out of your liver and lose half your body weight in a week. We are told to avoid carbohydrates, to stay away from meat, to only eat meat, to count our calories, to monitor our blood sugar – where will it end?

One of the keys to success is finding a new attitude to food and eating that is not about *dieting* but about *health*. Interestingly, there is very little disagreement about what a healthy diet really is. There is also no disagreement about what the modern diet is doing – it is killing us! One of the reasons that we keep eating the foods we are presented with in our local supermarkets and fast-food outlets is that we don't read the labels. We don't know what we are eating and many of us don't know how to cook.

The diet that we eat today in Europe and North America is a result of corporations placing profit over health. The primary focus of the food industry is to generate the maximum profit by producing foods that appeal to dramatic taste and convenience above any other considerations. This food has been made cheap largely by the application of government subsidies, to the extent that eating simple and unadulterated foods is often more expensive than eating fast foods. The true cost in terms of public health and environmental impact are not factored into the mix. The future of healthy nutrition will demand a much more comprehensive approach to the issue; to discover a healthy diet we need to consider several factors:

✿   **Potential toxicity**. This factor has to do with the way a certain food is used by the body – the way it contributes to a healthy internal environment or if it contains harmful elements that outweigh its benefits. Some individuals may be allergic to certain foods and those foods would be considered toxic, but many of us are exposed to substances in our food that are toxic by nature. These are usually chemicals that are used in food processing or in the growing of food.

✿   **Energy requirements and quantity**. Each of us is different in the way we digest, absorb and metabolize food. We also have different energy requirements: the needs of a nineteen-year-old elite athlete and a middle-aged office worker are going to be very different. A sedentary businessman who consumes the same diet as a Neolithic hunter is probably going to have problems. There are many foods that can provide nutritional stress if eaten too often or beyond actual need. A glass of wine might be nice once in a while; two or three glasses a day is a different matter.

✿   **Personal health needs**. As people learn more about food and its effects, they realize that they can change their diet in ways that provide certain health benefits. There are specific dietary adjustments that can help the body recover from illness. Chronic health problems – such as high blood pressure, diabetes, obesity and so many digestive disorders – are known to respond to specific dietary programs. Within the macrobiotic dietary system there are many individuals who have recovered from life-threatening diseases through the proper application of specific diets.

✿ **Climate and environment**. This consideration is central to some of the material contained in this book. Climate should be taken into account in any diet; to think that the body is immune or ignorant of these needs is a big mistake. The same rules apply to the changing seasons. Winters require foods that warm the body and give long-lasting energy – summer requires foods that aid cooling and relaxation. This is simply common sense.

✿ **Ecological impact**. For some people the issue of environmental impact of food selection may seem strange. We think of what we eat as an issue of nutrition not ecology, but nothing could be further from the truth. When people say that health is an issue of balance, we have to ask what we are balancing. In the final analysis, our health is a reflection of the way we create balance with our environment. As you will see in the following chapters, a diet that is healthy for an individual's health is also healthy for society and the planet. Sometimes the truth sounds magical, don't you think?

This chapter is all about the bad news. If you already know that there are hidden dangers in the modern diet, you can skip this chapter; if you are unconvinced or sitting on the fence, read on. Facts are facts.

The damage done by the contemporary diet falls into four categories of extreme consumption – chemicals, simple sugars, fat and protein. The misuse of these four components in our diet is the foundation of the health crisis we now face. We begin with the easiest to understand – chemicals.

The Chemical Cocktail

There are more than three thousand different chemical additives used in food processing. We are told that these chemicals are used to "enhance" the food, but it would be more accurate to say that they are used to disguise the food. We would not eat most of the food that is presented to us without it being chemically doctored – the color, taste and texture would otherwise be disgusting. To add insult to injury, many of these "enhancers" are known carcinogens.

Additives to Avoid

✿ **Artificial sweeteners**. Aspartame, marketed under the brand names NutraSweet and Equal, is believed to be carcinogenic and accounts for more reports of adverse reactions than all other foods and food additives put together.

✿ **High-fructose corn syrup (HFCS)**. This increases your low-density lipoprotein (LDL) cholesterol levels (or "bad" cholesterol levels) and contributes to the development of diabetes.

✿ **Monosodium glutamate (MSG)**. Used as a flavor enhancer, MSG is an excitotoxin, a substance that can overexcite and damage cells.

✿ **Trans-fats**. Numerous studies show that trans-fats increase LDL cholesterol levels and increase the risk of heart attacks, heart disease and strokes.

✿ **Common food dyes**. Artificial colorings may contribute to behavioral problems in children and have been implicated in significant reductions in IQ.

✿ **Sodium sulphite**. This is a preservative used in processed foods. People who are sulphite sensitive can experience headaches, breathing problems and rashes.

✿ **Sodium nitrate/nitrite**. This common preservative has been linked to various types of cancer.

✿ **Butylated hydroxyanisole (BHA) and butylated hydroxytoluene (BHT)**. BHA and BHT are preservatives that affect the neurological system, alter behavior and have the potential to cause cancer.

✿ **Sulphur dioxide**. Sulphur additives are toxic and in the United States they have been prohibited in raw fruit and vegetables. Adverse reactions include bronchial problems, low blood pressure and anaphylactic shock.

✿ **Potassium bromate**. An additive that is used to increase volume in some breads. It is known to cause cancer in animals, and even small amounts can create problems in humans.

It seems that the food industry feels that the issue with cancer-causing additives is not that they cause cell mutation, but how much we can tolerate before they kill us. I don't know about you but if something causes cancer or any health problem, I really don't want any of it. Allergic reactions, harm to infants and a variety of health problems are associated with our modern "chemical diet." The potential health risks of single chemical ingredients are amplified by the fact that no one knows what happens when they are all combined into the chemical cocktail that most people consume daily. This is especially true when we consider that the lists of additives do not include those chemicals that find their way into our vegetables from agricultural application. Yikes!

Some Additions to Your Vegetables

Fertilizers, herbicides and pesticides are the sources of many harmful chemicals introduced into the food chain. Fertilizers are used to produce larger and healthier-looking plants. Research has shown that the overuse of chemical fertilizers can reduce the nutritional content of food and that some seem to be harmful to the human reproductive system – oops.

✿ **Organophosphates**. A family of highly toxic pesticides that work by killing the brains and nervous systems of insects. Organophosphates are still widely used and have been found in disturbingly high quantities on many fruits and vegetables. Research has found that these chemicals can also harm the brains and nervous systems of human beings.

✿ **Dieldrin**. An organochlorine insecticide that, although now banned in the United States, is highly persistent and still present in many soils. Classified as a persistent organic pollutant (POP), it has the capacity to remain in the environment and in human body fat for long periods of time.

✿   **Methomyl**. A broad-spectrum insecticide from the carbamate group, used to control insects in a wide range of crops. As a carbamate, it works by inhibiting an enzyme essential for proper functioning of the nervous system. This acutely toxic insecticide is found in many fruits and vegetables. It is also a suspected endocrine disruptor and a potential groundwater contaminant.

✿   **Maleic hydrazide**. A herbicide used to prevent crops such as onions and potatoes from sprouting. It contains small quantities of hydrazine, a known toxin, which may leak into water reservoirs.

There has been a long battle to control pesticides. They are used to kill unwanted organisms, but who thinks that something that can kill one form of life is harmless to others? You may have noticed that pesticides come and go. A new one is used until it is found to be toxic to humans or domestic animals, and then it is banned and a newer one joins the ranks. Innocent till proven guilty seems a good policy in criminal proceedings, but it is a horrible way to approach public health. It amounts to an experiment conducted on society for commercial interests.

Avoiding chemicals in our diet is not really that difficult. Reading labels is one of the most useful things you can do; if the list of ingredients on the package is as long as your arm, it's probably not a good idea to eat that particular food. If there are any ingredients having more than three syllables, the food item in question was probably made in a laboratory. If the print is so small that you need a magnifying glass, or the list is cleverly tucked under a flap on the pack, you have to wonder what is being hidden.

The second wise choice is to support the growing of organic foods. Organic growers are sustaining a healthy environment and helping to save the most valuable resource we have – a living soil. Eating organic and locally grown fruits and vegetables is one of the best things we can do for the environment on a daily basis. Chemical additives and chemicals used in agriculture that find their way into our food are toxic and should be avoided as much as possible.

The Sweet Life

Sugar is another story. It seems impossible that there would be anyone who doesn't know that refined sugar is detrimental to health, and yet the consumption of simple sugars continues to rise. Part of the problem has to do with a basic misunderstanding about the fact that there are different kinds of sugars – some are harmful, some are good, some are better and some are best.

Simple Sugars

The term "sugar" refers to a class of crystalline carbohydrates, mainly *sucrose, lactose* and *fructose*, which are all sweet to the taste. However, "sugar" is often used as a word for sucrose, or simple sugar, which is normally used as a table condiment or in home cooking – it comes primarily from sugar cane or sugar beet. Other simple sugars are used in industrial food preparation, but are usually known by more specific names – *glucose, fructose* or fruit sugar, and high-fructose *corn syrup*. Simple sugars (monosaccharides and disaccharides) are rapidly absorbed into the body and quickly raise blood sugar levels. Here are some of the common simple sugars found in processed food:

✿   Fructose – found in honey and extracted from fruits

✿   Galactose – found in milk and dairy products

✿   Glucose – found in honey and fruits, but also extracted from vegetables

✿   Lactose – found in milk and made up of glucose and galactose

✿   Maltose – extracted from barley

✿   Sucrose – found in plants and made up of glucose and fructose

These simple sugars are found today in virtually all processed foods. They are used as flavoring agents and also as preservatives. Most people are unaware of their presence in a variety of common food items from baked goods to tomato paste and canned beans. Processed table sugar is a staple in most homes but has virtually no nutritional value left after processing. In fact, sugar has a negative nutritional value – we are less well nourished after using it than when not using it.

Simple sugars are absorbed into the body quickly, creating a spike in blood sugar levels and sometimes a quick burst of energy. The problem is that this sudden rise in blood sugar stimulates the pancreas to secrete insulin to lower the sugar level back to normal. When we use sugar regularly over the course of the day, our blood sugar rises and falls like a yo-yo. This puts stress on the pancreas that can lead to diabetes and a leaching of vitamins and minerals from the body, and is partly responsible for a number of physical and emotional imbalances. Overuse of simple sugars can contribute to feelings of stress, anxiety and even depression.

The late Dr. John Yudkin, Professor of Nutrition at London University, had this to say on the topic:

> *If only a small fraction of what is already known about the effects of sugar were to be revealed in relation to any other material used as a food additive, that material would promptly be banned.*
> *(Yudkin 1972)*

Since food companies know that some consumers are becoming "sugar savvy," they are trying to confuse the issue with a dishonest labeling policy. Ingredients such as sucrose, fructose and maltose may sound better to some people but if it ends in "ose" watch out! I have even seen an ingredient in America called "dried cane juice" – now, I wonder what that could be?

According to an article in the *British Medical Journal*, "Sugar is as dangerous as tobacco [and] should be classified as a hard drug, for it is harmful and addictive," and *The Guardian* (Thursday 15 February 2007) reports that "Sugars in all forms are seen by many as dangerous to health and our food is packed full of them: not just sucrose (plain sugar as we know it) but other forms of refined sugars from cane, beet and corn." Researchers from the Medical Research Council and the University of Cambridge (2007) developed a new urine test that allowed them to measure sugar consumption for the first time. They found that obese people dramatically underestimated the amount of sugar they consumed each day; those who ate the most consumed as much as 207 grams a day, hidden in everyday foods – that's nearly fifty-two spoonfuls and four times the recommended daily limit. It seems absurd but not when you figure that most fizzy drinks have between nine and fifteen teaspoons of sugar, or that a piece of white bread contains three teaspoons.

The body runs on carbohydrates – they are our primary source of energy. This is because they can be readily converted into glucose, the form of sugar that's transported and used by the body. The issue is where we get our carbohydrates and how easily the body can use them. *Simple carbohydrates*, or simple sugars, are extracted or exist in plants that may or may not be grown organically. Their effect on health is generally detrimental and they should be avoided or seldom used. *Complex carbohydrates*, or complex sugars, are preferred since they come combined with vitamins, minerals and essential buffering agents that aid their digestion and use. We will talk about complex (good) carbohydrates later (see page 46), but now it's time to move on to the next nutritional culprits in the modern diet – fat and protein.

The Animal Farm

You will notice that the recipes in this book are vegan, which means that there are no animal foods used. Eating this way is my choice and is what makes me feel good. My diet gives me great energy and vitality. Even as a child I was uncomfortable with the idea of eating animals. Some members of my family eat differently and so do many of my friends – it's their choice. I am not going to go into the moral aspects of using animal products here (that's for another book), but let me share with you some of the problems they pose to a healthy diet.

There is a mythology that humans evolved by eating meat and that it is our "natural food." This opinion is being seriously challenged by some recent scientific discoveries. Studies of Paleolithic cultures, as well as dietary investigation of the hunter-gatherer tribes remaining on the planet today, have shown that they consumed a varied diet that included vegetable-quality food, including undomesticated grains, wild plants and grasses, tubers, berries and roots.

"There was no one Stone Age diet; diets of the past varied greatly. People in Africa probably ate less meat than many people think," says John Gowlett, an archaeologist at Liverpool University, "while those in the northern, icy regions were forced to eat only whatever animals they could catch."

"I'm not convinced that we know what Stone Age man ate," agrees Andrew Millard, who researches ancient health and diet at Durham University. "The evidence we have is heavily biased towards the meat component of the diet. We get bones from animals they have eaten but we don't get the remains of any vegetables they have eaten because they decay. There is good evidence that later Stone Age cultures in the Near East regularly collected and ate wild cereals and it's possible the practice was more widespread" (*The Guardian*, Thursday 4 December 2003).

Our ideas about food are governed by many mythologies and the "meat for men" one is amusing. It made me smile when I thought about the woman who, at our last workshop, presented us with a newspaper article about why we should all eat red meat for good health! Well, of course, Bill and I checked out the study, which turned out to be bogus – no surprise there. A little research showed that the study was sponsored by an organization funded by several food companies. You need to be up early to catch me out on that one.

However, let's go back to the Paleolithic cultures. As little as 5 to 25% of their total food intake may have comprised fish and other sources of animal meat. These foods were eaten primarily when there was a lack of edible vegetation, or when tribes were on the move. In an article published in the Proceedings of the National Academy of Science, in October 2010, Anna Revedin, Jiri Svoboda and associates found convincing evidence that ancient diets were much different to what has always been assumed. Ancient humans during the Paleolithic Period and possibly even Neanderthals were using flour made from grains and starchy plants as a significant part of their diet. Our ancestors were baking biscuits 30,000 years ago!

In an article in Zeenews.com (2010), Revedin states,

> *Cooking enhances digestibility and also the taste of starch is improved by cooking.... We are quite convinced that flour enhanced [prehistoric humans'] mobility capacity, since it ensured a good source of energetic food during their travels.*

There is no doubt that milk, cheese and the meat of birds, fish and mammals as well as insects have played a part in the human diet. As society has changed, so has the food we eat – or it might be the other way around. Our ancestors moved out of their indigenous habitats and spread out in many directions. Human beings have lived in just about every environment from desert and tundra to mountaintops and tropical islands. As human populations moved, the diet had to adapt to different climate, soil, growing seasons and available flora and fauna. If we follow the thinking expressed above, what is being said is that we used animal products when they were essential to survival. They aren't anymore.

Saturated Fats and Disease

Approximately 30–35% of cancer cases are related to diet, physical inactivity and obesity. The World Cancer Research Fund (2011) has confirmed these figures. Excess body weight is associated with the development of many types of cancer and is a factor in 14–20% of all cancer deaths. Physical inactivity is believed to contribute to cancer risk not only through its effect on body weight, but also through negative effects on the immune and endocrine systems. Many of the most pressing health issues we face today are related to the overconsumption of animal fats and protein.

During the past century, dairy product consumption has risen sharply due to pasteurization and the increased ability to preserve and transport these products. In the past thirty years the idea that milk products are essential foods in a healthy diet has been proven to be wrong. Excessive consumption of highly saturated fat in dairy produce has been proven to contribute to heart disease and some cancers. These products include cheese, butter, milk (buttermilk, skimmed milk), yogurt, ice cream, cream, sour cream and whipped cream. They are all best left out of a healthy diet. The connection between dairy and meat consumption with cancer (primarily of the breast, bowel and stomach) is largely ignored.

A study by Boston's Harvard Medical School and Brigham and Women's Hospital (2003) was published in the *Journal of the National Cancer Institute*. The lead nutrition researcher, Enunyoug Cho, stated that a diet high in animal fat raised the risk of cancer by as much as 54%. This was a study of 90,000 women over an eight-year period, and is only one of an overwhelming number of studies arriving at the same conclusion.

Dr. T. Colin Campbell, the world's foremost epidemiological researcher and author of the best-selling book *The China Study* (2006) goes one step further. He believes that animal proteins are the prime carcinogen in meat and dairy products. He states that "human studies support the carcinogenic effect of animal protein, even at usual levels of consumption. … No chemical carcinogen is nearly so important in causing human cancer as animal protein."

Potential health risks of switching to a diet with little or no animal protein have been exaggerated beyond belief by the meat and dairy industries. According to the American Institute for Cancer Research and the World Cancer Research Fund, from their report on diet and cancer prevention (2009–11):

> *There is no essential lower limit of intake of any type of meat, and diets including no meat are not only compatible with good health and low cancer risk, but may be preferred in some settings, especially when plant foods are abundant, reliable and varied.*

Most people are aware of the connection between heart disease and diet. This is the number one health problem in the UK and United States today. My hometown, Glasgow, is now the "capital of disease" in Europe. Most heart disease is diet related – caused by diets high in animal products.

William Castelli, M.D., director of the Framingham Heart Study (2011) (the longest-running clinical study in medical history, beginning in 1948), says of the heart disease epidemic, "If we adopted a vegetarian diet, the whole thing would disappear." He has been threatened by McDonald's lawyers and repeatedly slammed by the meat and dairy industries, but Castelli refuses to back down. Americans have been "brainwashed to eat meat," he says, "and it's killing us." Not only do half of all Americans die of heart disease, but 80% of Americans will die *with heart disease in their body*. Once again, Castelli looks at the research – studies that go all the way back to 1904.

No plant food in the world contains cholesterol, but meat, eggs and dairy products contain high quantities of this fatty substance as well as high levels of saturated fat. When cholesterol builds up inside the walls of the arteries, the blood flow throughout the body is restricted. This restriction means that healthy bodily functions are impaired, contributing to a number of diseases, most notably heart disease. Both the fat and the protein in animal products can be a problem, but unfortunately the problem doesn't end there.

Growth Hormones and Antibiotics

Dairy foods and meat can come from animals that have been doped with hormones or other chemical additives in their food. In North America the use of growth hormones in cattle is still allowed, even though it is banned in the EU, but the debate still goes on. The use of rBGH (recombinant bovine growth hormone) finds its way into both milk and meat. These hormones become lodged in the fat tissue of animals, and the human consumption of these animals has been associated with some cancers as well as early disruption of sexual development in children.

In addition to hormones, the overuse of non-therapeutic antibiotics in poultry, beef cattle and swine production poses a serious threat to human health. Because half of these antibiotics belong to classes of drugs used in human medicine, the risk of antibiotic resistance in humans is increased. This is especially threatening to people with compromised immune systems, including infants, elderly people and cancer patients receiving chemotherapy. Antibiotic resistance in humans is a tremendous public health threat worldwide. With each generation, we have strayed further and further away from our roots in nature and have experienced a corresponding increase in chronic illness.

Food and the Environment

There is much concern about the effect that our modern lifestyle has on the environment. As we become more educated we want to lower our personal contributions to various forms of pollution – this is living with consciousness. We are all part of the web of life and need to respect that. Along with recycling and other valuable personal acts, the food we choose may have the greatest impact. Studies carried out by the U.N. Food and Agriculture Organization (FAO) in 2006 have indicated that reducing meat and dairy consumption may be the greatest individual act that a person can make towards a healthy planet.

In early 1971 Frances Moore Lappé first published her book *Diet for a Small Planet* (20th Anniversary Edition published in 1991). She brought into the public consciousness several important and urgent messages regarding food production and consumption. Among these was the fact that there is enough food to feed the hungry of the world if we use our crops with a greater degree of intelligence and social judgement. Some of these points were again put forward by John Robbins (1987) in his book *Diet for a New America*. Both of these fine books point to the need for a radical restructuring of our attitudes regarding agriculture, food consumption and distribution.

Part of the problem lies in our regard for food only as a product – something to be bought and sold. When we view food in this way it devalues it. Food must be approached with a special ethic in terms of its growth and use. This is especially true when we see that a small portion of the world's population is wasting food and literally eating itself to death, while the remainder of the world is dying of starvation and malnutrition. Acting against the creative flow of life in nature produces economic chaos, sickness and death. It is an outcome that must be clearly understood, not as a punishment, but as the result of our lack of wisdom and an abuse of our freedom. If we do not change our relationship to the foods we eat, not only will we suffer poor individual health, but the impact of our choices will affect society and the environment as well.

One of the benefits of Living with the Seasons is that it naturally promotes a more ecological way of eating. What you may discover is that when we eat a diet that is healthy for us, it just so happens to be one that is sustainable and produces the least waste and pollution. But why would we be surprised? If everything in nature is connected, then health must mean being in concert with nature, not disruptive to it.

In the next chapter I am going to take you back in time thousands of years and explore how many cultures all over the world understood the puzzle of life and health. Inside many of these ancient systems lie gems of wisdom that are just as valuable today as they were then. The lessons of natural cycles in the world around us are reflected in the internal workings of the body. These are the lessons of Living with the Seasons and they are there for all of us to use and enjoy.

What I have done is interpret the wisdom of cultures around the world to develop a practical and effective method to create health. I have built this approach on the folk traditions of Asia, with influences from Europe and the Americas. The reason that these ways of thinking are important is that they represent the history of human inquiry into how to maintain health. The cycle of the seasons, most beautifully expressed in Chinese medicine, is helpful since it represents a highly sophisticated view of human ecology. The Chinese understood that the organ systems of the body as well as the mind and spirit must conform to natural cycles of the year to maintain good health. It may be fascinating to know that much of what was written thousands of years ago aligns with the most recent nutritional research. First, we need to understand the logic of this approach before looking at how that way of thinking can be applied to modern life.

Chapter 4

HEALTHY FOOD

When I was recovering from a serious accident many years ago, I started paying even more attention to what I ate and began to study more about nutrition. I didn't want to become a nutritionist or overly focused on diet, but what I began to read really opened my eyes. When we notice that some cultures are slender and have a much lower rate of degenerative disease, shouldn't that be telling us something? There is a mountain of scientific evidence indicating that the healthiest diet you can consume is one that is high in complex carbohydrates, vegetables and plant proteins. Many studies have shown that if people eat this way, heart disease and diabetes are reversed and a plethora of chronic diseases prevented. What do they eat? Well, they eat the kind of wholefood, plant-based diet that you are going to learn about.

There is a lot of concern regarding the value of different foods in a healthy diet and the quality of the foods we eat. There are serious questions about the chemicals that have found their way onto our plates. This "chemical cocktail" is composed of fertilizer and pesticide residues, hormones pumped into meat, and the thousands of chemical additives used to flavor, texture, color and preserve the food we eat. Yum yum. These are non-nutritive and often toxic additions to our food – and our body doesn't know what to do with them.

When I teach Living with the Seasons cooking classes (which are a lot of fun), clients are absolutely amazed with the results they achieve in a short period of time. Whether they want to detox their system or lose weight, or are looking for relief from symptoms they have lived with for years, they can see the difference. They feel more alive, have increased energy and sleep better.

Many of the spouses of students I have taught try these new dishes with trepidation and I know what is coming ... I know what they are going to say before they even speak. I can voice it alongside them. "Hmmm, well, it's OK. Actually it's quite tasty. In fact this is very good and you say it has sea vegetables in it?" ... "I would never have believed it could taste this good!" It warms the cockles of my wee heart when another family comes on board, eating these incredible healing foods.

Every day, we choose what to purchase and what to eat. I will present my version of the Asian system of understanding in a way that respects personal tastes and backgrounds, with recipes that reflect a fusion of both Oriental and European influences. To do this I use two approaches: the first one is the theory of the five tastes, which comes from China; the second is the macrobiotic system, from Japan. These are wonderful ways to cook with variety and imagination.

One of the reasons that many people fail when they try to change their diet is that they may have cravings. These cravings have many sources, one of which is simply to create a balance of taste. We are aware of this when we eat something salty and immediately want a drink, but generally this process is not quite so dramatic. In Traditional Chinese Medicine (TCM) the five tastes are used to completely satisfy our desires. The tastes are known to not only affect the flavor of the food but also stimulate the function of different organs in the body and supply different kinds of energy to our lives. Practically speaking, the more you consciously include a variety of the five tastes in food preparation, the more satisfying and nutritionally enhanced your meals will be. The result is a reduction in cravings.

Of course, some cravings are simply there because we want to feel differently. Examples of such substances include alcohol, sugar, salt, coffee and chocolate. These foods change our body chemistry and result in a change in behavior or perception. Eating a carrot is not going to make you want to dance on the table, but a few glasses of champagne might. The five-taste program is designed to change your palate and to provide alternatives so that your body is no longer interested in the extra sugar, salt, sweets, coffee or chocolates. (This doesn't mean you might not feel like having a glass of bubbly when the mood takes you.)

My aim is to redress the balance so as to create health that satisfies taste in a way that is comfortable and sustainable. Many people's taste buds have long since been spoiled by chemicals used as flavoring agents and by excessively refined sugars, so much so that to appreciate the natural sweetness of a carrot or onion is completely alien.

My own diet is 100% plant based. That means I eat a variety of grains and beans; a wide range of vegetables, sea vegetables, fruits, seeds and nuts; and some of the soy protein foods that originate in the Orient. I don't expect everyone to eat like me (though I wish they did), but the basic facts are hard to ignore.

I have miso soup every day. This delicious soup, made from the fermented paste of soybeans, has become a health ritual in my kitchen. I introduce it to everyone I teach and they always thank me. I figure that if the healthiest nation in the world eats it daily, then it's on my menu. The latest studies on miso demonstrate its incredible powers of disease prevention. This is something that was known in the Far East hundreds of years before the advent of nutritional science. It is important that we start to respect and learn from many of these old traditions.

When I am teaching there is often a sense of frustration from the students or clients at our workshops. They wonder why they have never been presented with the kind of information and simple-living techniques described in this book. They tell me that they feel lighter, calmer and "clean inside," to name but a few, when they eat this way. They wonder why their doctor hasn't told them to change their diet or to get more exercise – I wonder why too. I suppose it comes down to the fact that the members of the medical establishment are so focused on sickness that they have no time for health.

Many of our attitudes about health come from questionable sources with conflicting agendas. In fact, advertising is a major source of health information. That is a scary reality; advertising is about profit, not progress. My wildest dream would be to see wonderful advertisements on TV for natural foods, instead of being bombarded with advertisements about fizzy drinks or hamburgers.

Foods to Use Regularly for Better Health

Whole-Cereal Grains

Since the beginning of human development of agriculture, cereal grains have been the principal food for humanity. In Europe, Asia, Africa and the Americas, grain has always been the staple food. The advantage of whole grains is that they have a broad range of nutrients as well as fiber. They also combine well with other vegetable-quality foods to provide the best variety for human nutritional needs.

It is only in the past seventy years that diets in the affluent countries have seen a decrease in the consumption of whole grains and an increase in meat, dairy and refined foods: a change that has contributed greatly to most of the degenerative diseases in modern society. Wholegrain rice, barley, oats, kasha, rye, quinoa and varieties of wheat are all members of the grain family.

Because grains can feed the largest number of people per acre and are easily stored, they are ideal from ecological and economical points of view. Try to buy grains that are produced in your climatic zone for the least environmental impact. Your recipes should include many grain dishes. Even though it is best to use whole grains, variety can be achieved by including partially refined grains or flours in your diet as well.

Wholegrain flour products lack some of the nutritional value of whole grains but are useful for naturally fermented breads or other baked products. Grinding breaks the outer shell of the grain, leading to oxidation and loss of nutritional value. The same holds true for wholegrain flakes. Although these foods are useful for added variety, it is best to focus on whole grains for the foundation of your diet.

Refined flour, such as white flour, has many of the same problems as refined sugar. Since it is fragmented and has some of the nutrients removed, it lacks the nutritional density found in whole grain. White-flour products are difficult to digest and often lead to digestive stagnation and weight gain. Despite having some of their nutrition removed, if used sparingly, items such as refined rice, bulgur wheat, couscous and polenta are a nice addition for extra variety in the diet.

A large-scale shift away from these traditional staples began with the Industrial Revolution and coincided with the rise of modern degenerative disease. The largest proportion of protein in the modern diet comes from meat, eggs, poultry, dairy products and other animal sources. Most of the fat is saturated animal fat rather than polyunsaturated vegetable oil; and, whereas in the past people based their diets on unrefined complex carbohydrates (such as whole grains, beans, and vegetables), people today consume carbohydrates primarily in the form of refined grains and simple sugars.

A balanced diet of whole grains, beans and vegetables produces a calming and centering effect on the body and mind and relaxes feelings of tension or pressure. Eating well is the long-term answer to stress. The complex carbohydrates or polysaccharides in whole grains exist together with an ideal balance of minerals, proteins, fats and vitamins. These complex sugars are gradually and smoothly assimilated through the digestive organs, providing the body with a slow and steady source of energy. Cereal grains find their home in most traditional diets in wholegrain products, porridge, breads, noodles, and a variety of crackers and other baked items. The best nutritional use of grain is as whole grain – it is easier to digest than flour products.

The whole-cereal grains include barley, maize, millet, oats, whole (brown) rice, rye, sorghum, spelt, teff, triticale, wheat and wild rice. Two seeds that are usually included in this category, but are not botanically grains, are quinoa and buckwheat (kasha).

Vegetables

Fresh vegetables, rich in a wide range of vitamins, minerals and antioxidants, are an essential part of a healthy diet. Since many vegetables begin to lose nutritional content once picked, it is important that they are used as fresh as possible. A good diet contains a variety of vegetables defined by shape, color, season of growth and nutritional content.

Because vegetables vary in the degree of perishability, it is important to use them in the season of growth. This is a principle of eating with the seasons. Vegetables that grow in the spring and summer are generally more perishable than root vegetables and ground vegetables that ripen in the autumn or early winter. As you will see in the recipes, we try to eat easily perishable foods when they are ready to eat and save the more hearty ones for later consumption. This is the best pattern to follow.

Vegetables can be eaten either cooked or raw. You will notice in the recipes that the summer and spring meals feature more raw or lightly cooked vegetables. In the winter we use vegetables that are harder to digest when eaten raw, and need the cooking to release all the energy of the food and produce a more warming effect. In the recipe sections there are also several instructions on how to make simple pickles at home in a short time – pickling creates useful enzymes that aid digestion.

In our classification system we generally group vegetables according to their qualities and not their botanical family. The most common categories we use are (i) hearty greens, (ii) light greens and summer vegetables, (iii) ground vegetables and (iv) root vegetables.

Hearty greens include kale, broccoli, collard greens, spring greens, Swiss chard, napa cabbage, beet leaves, dandelion greens, carrot tops and turnip greens. These vegetables generally grow late in the season and often have a slightly bitter taste if eaten raw and contain a higher concentration of minerals than the summer greens.

Examples of **light greens and summer vegetables** are asparagus, spinach, beet leaves, celery, bok choy (Chinese cabbage, also known as *pak choi*), endive, lettuce, nettles, alfalfa or bean sprouts, romaine lettuce and arugula. These greens are generally used in the spring and summer and have a cooling and expansive effect when eaten. Green beans, runner beans and various sprouted beans, such as mung bean, as well as other sprouts belong to this group too.

Ground vegetables are generally harvested in the autumn and early winter and include cauliflower, green cabbage, white cabbage, hard-skinned squash and vegetable marrow (green summer squash). Some varieties of squash are easy to store through the winter months and include Hubbard squash, butternut squash, acorn squash and pumpkin. These vegetables are excellent when cooked with beans or in vegetable stews, and can be warming; also, when baked, they are very sweet. (*Note*: The yellow variety of summer squash, zucchini and cucumbers are usually used in summer or late summer).

Root vegetables are used all year round, but more commonly in the winter. They are easily stored and have a warming, contracting energy. Carrot, parsnip, turnip, yam, radish, sweet potato and the Japanese daikon radish (called *mooli* in some Asian shops) are all roots. I have included burdock root in some recipes: it is increasingly found in natural foods markets in the UK and America and is a wonderful mineral-rich addition to the winter cupboard.

Beans and Bean Products

Proteins form the major solid matter of our muscles, organs, glands, bones, teeth, skin, nails and hair. Protein, in fact, is necessary for the building and repairing of all body tissues. Proteins are made up of twenty-two building blocks, called *amino acids*. Nine amino acids are designated *essential* because the body cannot produce them – they must be absorbed from the food we eat. Animal proteins contain all of the essential amino acids. However, animal protein can cause the body to become over-acidic, and commercially grown meat is high in saturated fat.

Plant proteins have different combinations of amino acids which, when combined from various sources (i.e. grain, bean, nut and seed), complement each other and are considered "complete" proteins. These complementary proteins do not have to be combined at the same meal, because the body stores amino acids and then draws upon these reserves to make the protein complete.

Beans have served as a natural complement to a grain-based diet for centuries in Asia, Africa, Europe and both North and South America. Among the most popular varieties are red kidney beans, garbanzos (chickpeas), pinto beans, adzuki beans, lentils (red, brown and green varieties), lima beans, and a wide variety of dried peas and beans. Out of all these, the soybean is the one most referred to because of its high protein content and is often thought of as a replacement for meat or dairy in the diet. A variety of "health food" products in the form of soy cheese, soy milk and a range of imitation meat products made from soy (such as vegan sausages, cutlets and burgers) are on the market. However, the usefulness of these products is questionable: the problem is that soy is difficult to digest. This can be true of all beans if they are not cooked well, but the soybean is particularly stubborn.

For centuries soy has been used as a staple of the Asian diet. In fact it is seen as one of the most important health benefits of the Chinese and Japanese way of eating. Soy was tamed by fermenting the beans to make a variety of delicious and tasty products that actually increase the benefits of the soybean. Products such as miso, soy sauce, tempeh and natto are all fermented and easier to digest. Tofu is not fermented but is used modestly in traditional use. Soy milk and other raw soy products are very difficult to digest and are not a great choice, especially for the very young.

Miso is a fermented bean paste that provides a wide variety of enzymes and bacteria which are beneficial to the digestive system and aid in food absorption. Miso also contains proteins, vitamins and minerals and is one of the world's most medicinal foods. The daily use of miso can lower cholesterol and balance the blood's pH. Miso may include grain as well as soybeans and is aged from eighteen months to two years.

Miso has been touted for centuries as a folk remedy for cancer, weak digestion, tobacco poisoning, low libido and several types of intestinal infections. Recently, scientists in Japan, China and the United States (Hirayama 1981; Ito 1989; Messina and Barnes 1991) have discovered that miso really is effective against atomic radiation, heavy metal poisoning, cardiovascular disease, many forms of cancer, strokes, high blood pressure, chronic pain and food allergies. Miso is a good source of some minerals and B vitamins, and its amino acids are well balanced by grains such as brown rice.

Shoyu and **tamari** are two types of soy sauce and excellent flavor enhancers. The essential difference between these two sauces is that tamari is wheat free. Both are natural and aged in cedar wood kegs for up to two years, and have no flavorings, colorings or preservatives added.

Tempeh is a pressed soybean cake, made from split soybeans, water and a special enzyme. This food is excellent to use in a variety of ways and is easy to cook and digest.

Natto is made from whole cooked soybeans, fermented using beneficial enzymes, and served with whole grains. It is also used in soups with vegetables.

Tofu, a fresh soybean curd, is made from soybeans and nigari (a natural sea salt coagulant) and used in small quantities in soups, vegetable dishes and dressings. Dried tofu can also be used in soups and vegetable dishes.

Studies (Hirayama 1971; Messina and Barnes 1991) have shown that soy has protective qualities for everyone, including breast cancer survivors, and that the fear of soy much written about in the media is unfounded (no surprise there!). Isoflavones, or plant estrogens, in soy have anti-cancer effects in both cell culture and animal studies. Furthermore, in Asian countries, where fermented soy is a staple food, the rates of breast cancer have traditionally been very low compared to those in the United States or Europe.

Research for the U.S. Department of Agriculture (USDA) conducted by Dr. James Duke (1999) and published in the *Journal of Alternative Complementary Medicine* has shown that fermentation of soybeans increases their isoflavone levels by a factor of 25 to 30. This research has been confirmed in Japan (Yamamoto 2002). The central issue is the fermentation: unfermented soy food is hard to digest and not a healthy option, but fermented soy products are beneficial.

Fermented soy foods, such as miso, soy sauce (e.g. shoyu and tamari) and natto miso, have twenty-five times more isoflavones compared to unfermented soy foods, such as tofu and soy milk. Also, when it comes to lowering cholesterol, a bowl of miso soup made with seaweed and shitake mushrooms is much more effective than either tofu or soy milk. And fermented soy foods have much lower levels of substances called *anti-nutrients* that can inhibit digestion of important nutrients.

Protein is a nutritional requirement, but it does make a difference where it comes from. One fact is becoming very clear: most people in modern society are eating too much animal-source protein. Another source of protein, and the nutritional companion to whole-cereal grains, in most cultures has traditionally been the legume. Beans supply some of the essential amino acids that grains lack and are a perfect addition to a diverse diet.

Sea Vegetables

Sea vegetables have been used in many parts of the world as a supplemental food and are a rich source of many trace minerals. They have ten to twenty times more mineral content than vegetables grown on land; these minerals include calcium, magnesium, potassium, iodine, iron and zinc.

In Japan, sea vegetables have been used to the best effect in soups and stews, and as side dishes and condiments. Sea vegetable foods are consumed in small portions and are becoming more readily available from European and North American sources. In the recipe sections you will see them used in soups and stews, bean dishes and even salads.

Sea vegetables are capable of binding with heavy metals and radioactive toxins in the body to safely escort them out. What is more, the minerals in sea vegetables exist in a chelated colloidal form that makes them readily bioavailable. When my dentist found an amalgam filling underneath an old crown that was being replaced, he had me take some chlorella before he proceeded. Now *that's* holistic dentistry.

The longevity and health of the people of Okinawa are believed to be due in part to their regular consumption of sea vegetables. Over the last few decades, medical researchers have discovered that a diet rich in sea vegetables reduces the risk of some diseases and helps the body eliminate toxins (Yamamoto et al. 1974).

There are many foods that are not commonly used in our culture but are widely used in others where there are thousands of years of experience of eating a simple, healthy and semi-vegetarian diet. Sea vegetables are an intelligent addition for health and longevity, along with fermented foods such as miso and naturally fermented soy sauce.

There is a long tradition of pickling vegetables in Europe and America. Nowadays, these foods are only seen as special condiments, but they once played an important function in traditional diets. Once we know how to use them, they provide incredible benefits and can be used in a wide variety of delicious dishes. As I mentioned earlier, as a teenager I discovered kelp seaweed and since then have been a user of these incredible healing plants from the sea.

Fruits

Fruits in small quantities are an important element of a healthy diet. It is best to select fruits that are grown in the local environment as a first choice. They may be used raw or in cooked desserts. Most fruits are naturally low in fat, sodium and calories. Beneficial fiber, minerals, antioxidants and vitamins, including folic acid (an important B vitamin), are all found in abundance in most fruit.

Since most fruits are quite perishable, I focus on trying to eat fruits in season and using those that grow in the climate where I live. This is the easiest approach to achieving a balanced diet. This means that fruit is eaten more in the summer and late summer, when the positive relaxing, cooling and expansive effects of these foods are more pronounced. The natural drying or canning of cooked fruits or jams for later use is quite common when not sugar sweetened.

Nuts and Seeds

Nuts and seeds are an excellent source of healthy oils and help to complement grains and beans for the full range of amino acids needed to meet protein requirements and the metabolism of many vitamins. Seeds are the better choice since the oils are easier to digest. For example, sunflower, pumpkin and sesame seeds are great if lightly roasted (roasting brings out the flavor) and sprinkled on breakfast porridge or used as a garnish on grain dishes.

With nuts it is best to use those that are grown in the climatic zone where we live. In the more moderate four-seasons climate, nuts such as hazel nuts, walnuts and almonds are good choices. The more tropical varieties – for instance Brazil nuts, macadamia nuts and cashews – are quite oily and more difficult to digest; these can be used, but in moderation.

Fats and Oils

The oils I use are all sourced from seeds, nuts or grains. Fats and oils act as major structural components in the membranes which surround the body's trillions of cells. As well as having important functions in the building and maintenance of healthy cells, they are an important source of energy for the body. Fats and oils are divided into two main types: *saturated* and *unsaturated*.

Saturated fats are found mostly in animal products. These fats tend to stick together and are deposited in the cells, organs and arteries, where they can harden. If eaten to excess, this clumping of saturated fats causes numerous health problems in both the digestive system and the circulatory system.

Unsaturated fats are found mostly in nuts, seeds and grains. These fats are fluid in the body and essential for body repair. They allow the molecules within the cell membranes to make and break contact with one another as they fulfil their important chemical and transport functions. Many vitamins are oil soluble and so are not used effectively if the body is deficient in good-quality oils.

Vegetable oils, such as sesame oil and olive oil, are an excellent source of dietary fats and an essential part of cooking. Choose the best-quality cold-pressed oils and use them in moderation.

A Pinch of Salt

Many professional chefs will tell you that there is only one proper seasoning – salt. Salt has been used for centuries to preserve, pickle and bring out the flavor of foods. The use of salt in prehistoric times liberated people from the seasons; by using salt to preserve and pickle foods, it became possible to keep fish, meats and vegetables through the winter. Salt also has the unique ability to bring out the flavor of many vegetable foods and whole grains.

Salt has gained a bad reputation over the last two decades as being potentially dangerous, but it is an important part of a healthy diet. Obviously having too much salt is not a good thing, but there is a difference between natural sea salt and refined table salt. Natural sea salt contains nearly sixty trace minerals, including sodium chloride, iodine and potassium. This salt can be used in moderation in cooking (not as a table condiment). Ordinary table salt that is bought in supermarkets has been stripped of its companion elements and contains additive elements such as aluminium silicate (a toxic element) to keep it powdery and porous. One of the problems is that people eating a diet of prepared foods often take in huge amounts of salt that is included as an ingredient. You don't have to worry, however, about the salt portions in my recipes.

Other herbs and spices are useful flavoring agents to complement the tastes of your ingredients. Common herbs and spices are often moderately used as flavoring agents, but you will notice that they are seldom used in seasonal cooking. I like to let the foods speak for themselves. Small amounts of basil and other garden herbs, as well as bay, ginger, garlic and simple spices, are used in moderation.

A Word about Water

No water, no life. We don't often think about water as a nutrient but it is the most important ingredient in our food. You can go for days without food, but don't try to go without water. It is the fundamental property of life and vital to all body functions, including movement, digestion and temperature regulation. Around 80% of our body weight is water: it is essential for metabolic functions, the transport and burning of fat, and the elimination of toxins from the body.

It is important to use the purest water available for drinking, cooking and bathing to prevent the absorption of pesticide residues, heavy metals (including lead from old plumbing) and chlorine. Rather than using bottled water, invest in a good water filter. Get one that has a carbon block, activated carbon filter and/or ceramic filter. Avoid reverse osmosis since it takes the minerals out of the water. You want to remove as many chemicals as possible, including the chlorine, but leave the minerals alone.

With the simplest healthy ingredients, together with some good recipes for reference and a spirit of adventure, you can create food that is healthy and delicious.

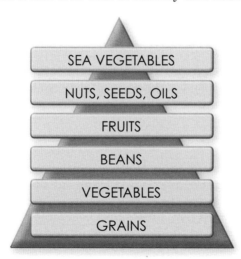

The food pyramid is one way of showing relative values of different food groups. At the bottom of the pyramid are the foods most used by volume. This may change depending on the season of the year or personal need or preference.

Chapter 5

LIFE ENERGY

Imagine that living is like floating down a river on a raft. Sometimes the water runs calm and slow, and sometimes it picks up pace and races down the rapids. Now imagine two ways of dealing with this river: one would be to constantly resist the stream, and the other would be to consciously move with it. According to the ancient Chinese philosophers who developed the Taoist philosophy – either we live within the laws of nature or we break them. Living within the laws of nature was seen to be the path to creating a healthy and happy life; breaking them was the path to sickness. This is a fairly simple concept and in no way takes away free will or the fact that sometimes we need to guide our raft over to the shore and walk for a while to avoid a waterfall.

Understanding these laws of nature was the task that the ancient sages set out to tackle. They didn't have the equipment that a modern scientist has at their disposal, but they were just as committed. They continued their studies for hundreds of years and came up with some wonderful discoveries and insights. Many of their ideas resonate with modern ideas in the area of health and diet. The more esoteric application of these principles described a very monastic way of life. The version we present is a very simplified interpretation that can be used with a specific focus on health. These ideas are thousands of years old, yet still have a practical application.

Western science has focused on the material aspects of cell functioning, tissue groupings, organ systems and gross anatomy; it is the study of detail. The Eastern approach placed more emphasis on attempting to understand the relationships of the parts to the whole; it is holistic and ecological. This more primitive approach to health was aimed at creating a balance between the individual and the environment. The guiding idea was to perceive the rules of nature and to follow them in daily life.

These two approaches are not necessarily mutually exclusive – in fact, they can be complementary. The only problem is that the practitioners of holism sometimes claim they are more enlightened, while the scientists say, "My way or the highway." I represent a third choice – use what works and rely on common sense.

Yin and Yang – The Pulse of Life

I like the macrobiotic approach to the classification of food presented by the Japanese philosopher George Ohsawa, who simplified the Chinese system and made it more user-friendly. Two concepts are central to his classification and these derive from the ancient philosophy of Taoism. They are based on the simple observation that there is a rhythmic movement in the way that nature works. This system is called *yin and yang*.

The basic theory of yin and yang simply states that energy pulsates and that this pulsation has two directions of movement – expansion and contraction. They observed that these patterns of movement were present in all of nature. In the body this is seen in the expansion and contraction of the muscles of the body; the rhythmic movements of the heart, lungs and intestines; and the flow of blood from the heart to the periphery and back again. All of nature operates according to this simple law, from the pulse of the galaxy to the throbbing of the smallest cell. The way in which nutrients are absorbed by the cells and the toxins released also reflects this tidal surge of yin and yang.

One of the applications of this way of viewing the life process was that certain foods produced or promoted a more contractive or expansive result in the body. The goal was to use foods in a way that produced harmony between these influences. The contractive force generates more heat, solidity and activity, while the expansive force creates a cooler, relaxed and dispersed energy. This influence is reflected in both body and mind – we still say that some people are "uptight," while others are "spaced-out." The list below gives some examples of common foods classified according to the contractive or expansive effect they have on the body.

Contractive foods (yang)	Expansive foods (yin)
Root vegetables	Leafy greens
Lentils and many dried beans	Green beans, runner beans
Seeds	Nuts
Whole grains	Refined grains
Salt	Sugar
Cheese	Milk
Meat	Fruit
	Food additives

Macrobiotic practitioners believe that certain characteristics of plants (and animals too) give a clue as to how they affect us when they are eaten. This effect is contained within the food and a result of the season it grows in and the environment of its growth, as well as qualities such as the taste, color and texture of the plant.

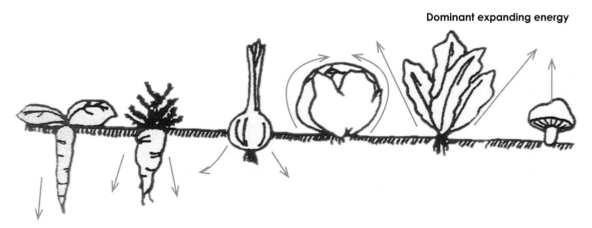

Dominant expanding energy

Dominant contracting energy

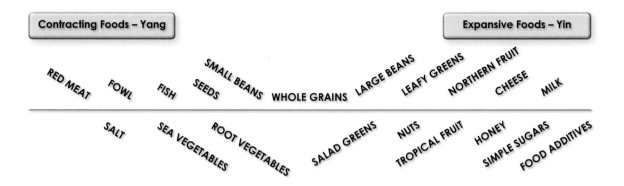

A partial list of foods from yang to yin. At the extremes, the effects of the food become unpredictable and so need more care in their use.

The macrobiotic approach focuses on choosing foods that produce the maximum nutrition with the least amount of stress on the digestive system, and the body's ability to efficiently use the nutrients. Foods that lie within the central range are generally considered to be more healthful and the best ones for daily use. It is recommended to reduce or avoid the foods lying at the extremes.

The Theory of the Five Transformations

The study of yin and yang energy is useful but is complemented in TCM by the theory of the Five Transformations. The dynamic interaction between yin and yang does not produce a universe of simply black and white. Because of the infinite possibilities of yin and yang interaction, each with varying degrees of dominance, a wide variety of energetic qualities is possible. This is just like the water of a river that changes its character dramatically from rapids to waterfalls to silent ponds, before eventually flowing into the sea. The primary energy of nature expresses itself with incredible diversity, but it is the appearance that changes and not the primary reality of the water.

Each season of the year is represented by an energy that dominates. Spring is dominated by *TREE* energy that rises and is the birthing of vegetal life. Summer is represented by *FIRE* – the energy of the sun and the season of abundance. As the energy of the summer wanes there is a swing season, late summer, when energy starts to settle – this is the time of *SOIL*. Autumn is ruled by *METAL* energy, when energy concentrates and settles into the earth. This settling and contracting energy is coiled and then released into *WATER*, the energy that animates winter before rising to continue the cycle.

The concept of seasonal eating is a basic principle in traditional health care systems from around the world. The truth is that people didn't use to have much of an option. When you don't have refrigerators and developed transportation systems, you eat what grows when it grows and learn to naturally preserve it, or you find out which foods can be safely stored.

One of the reasons that more people are drawn to this way of eating is that it supports regional self-sufficiency. If we can eat the foods that are produced closer to home it is better for the environment. Another reason to let the seasons guide us in food choices is that it is healthier. With enough flexibility to make a varied diet, the seasons give us what we need and serve as a guide for better health choices.

Our bodies reflect the history of our species; we are a walking reflection of how we have developed over the centuries. Sometimes we seem reluctant to admit it, but it's true. When the weather is hot, the body craves foods that cool us down; when it is cold, we want foods that warm us up. We may think that such considerations are silly, but we ignore the seasons at our own risk. Sometimes I see people walking down the street in winter with an ice cream and it makes me shiver. What must their poor body be feeling?

Each season presents specific challenges to the body, which requires specific nourishment for abundant health throughout the year. This system reflects the cycles of growth in nature and is part of a concept of human health that is ecological in perspective. To make the system easier, I use a modern interpretation of this ancient tradition that takes into account contemporary tastes and cultural preferences.

Modern technology has made it possible for us to eat seasonal foods at any time of year through the use of transportation, refrigeration and chemical preservation. This has of course provided the benefit of variety, but it has also lead to the denaturing of our food and the increased use of harmful chemicals. Our work is aimed not at turning back the clock, but rather at increasing personal awareness and controlling health. When we eat foods that have been transported, there is invariably a destructive effect on the environment. It is also true that the increasing popularity of many foods in modern society means that people in third-world countries lose their ability to grow food for themselves in order to provide exotic products for export to the wealthy consumer market.

The classifications of SOIL, METAL, WATER, TREE and FIRE are descriptions of qualitative changes in energetic transformation, which occur in the process of yin changing to yang and yang changing to yin. To use an example from nature, vegetation decays and is compressed over the centuries to become coal, which is then mined as a source of energy. This is burned to produce electricity, which is then consumed or used to produce new goods or services. Where did this process begin? Was it with the mining of the coal? Or was it with the growing of the plant?

In terms of the relationship between chi and physical function, the energies described in the theory of the Five Transformations provide the primal nourishment for the life process. In various forms, they combine to create the food we eat, the water we drink, the air we breathe and the radiation from the sun. Aside from the material nourishment, these five energies also have a profound effect on the vitality of our life process.

Stages of the Energy Cycle

The five stages should be seen as a sequence of events that moves in a continuing cycle. The terms used to describe these qualities are SOIL, METAL, WATER, TREE and FIRE. These terms should not be interpreted in the literal sense, but they do describe analogies that exist between these natural phenomena and the energetic qualities being discussed. Later, an attempt will be made to translate these analogies into a physical framework, but it is necessary to first put forward an image of each progressive stage as it occurs in nature.

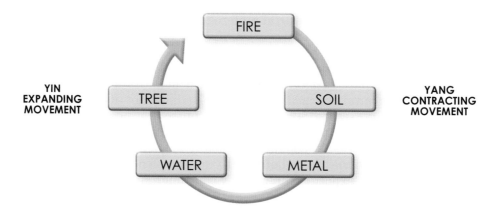

Energy moves from yin to yang and back again.

✿   **SOIL** – This energy can be seen as the first stage of contracting energy (yang). SOIL is energy that is settling, condensing and becoming more solid and contains the potential for everything material. The components for all matter are there, but in what could be described as the "soft" state. At this stage of yang, the contractive energy still has some malleable qualities. The image of the forest floor, where all matter is decomposed and broken down into constituents, is one that is often used. The top of the soil is soft and decaying, and rich in life and activity. As it settles deeper, it becomes more concentrated and firm. This settling process leads to the next stage of transformation – METAL.

✿   **METAL** – This stage is the most completely yang of the five stages. METAL is the extreme state of contraction and the stage of complete materialization where energy is most compact and tightly composed. An image often associated with this stage of energy is ore or stone. Because of the level of concentration described in this stage of transformation, there is a strong quality of energetic potential. Energy that reaches the ultimate stage of contraction seeks release and movement. Having reached the extremes of one pole, the tendency is then to return to the opposite – it moves to WATER.

✿ **WATER** – This describes the first energetic stage towards yin or expansion. The image of WATER indicates the more viscous qualities inherent in the beginnings of this movement and is the stage of energetic release, fluid in its movement. These energetic qualities are clearly seen by observation of water in the environment. Rain falls upon the earth and flows into lakes, rivers and streams, moving continually towards the sea, where it evaporates and ascends back to the atmosphere in a never-ending cycle towards and then away from the earth. The movement of water in its stage of evaporation is closely aligned with the energetic qualities described in the next energy – TREE energy.

✿ **TREE** – This describes energy that is ascending – the impulse behind the growth of plants upwards and towards the sun, the rising energy of morning mists, and any movement up and away from the surface of the planet. TREE energy is a further progression of the yin or expansive tendencies of water, but it is more controlled or channelled; it has a more defined direction of movement. This energy moves with what could be described as a directness of purpose, in a more ordered and defined fashion. Just like a sprouting seed moving towards the sun, TREE energy moves towards FIRE.

✿ **FIRE** – The image of this stage is analogous to the sun itself. FIRE is the plasmic and fiery energy of combustion – the great transformation between the yin and yang phases of the energetic cycle. It produces warmth that radiates out from itself, but consumes and diminishes its very substance. FIRE energy encompasses the most extreme polarities and qualities of all the stages of transformation. It manifests extreme yin in its radiant powers, which can then begin the slow condensation back into SOIL, reducing energy to its refined basis. But it also contains within it the yang qualities of condensation and breaks down that which it consumes.

Each phase of development in this transformation cycle is essential to the next. The effectiveness of energy in manifesting itself in each successive phase depends upon how effectively the energy has reached its full potential in the preceding phase. In order for a complete condensation of yang energy in METAL, there must be an adequate resource of SOIL. In order for the potential to be released into the questing qualities of WATER, METAL must have consolidated its resources to the maximum. In order for TREE energy to have the upward lift and lightness that is its potential, there must be the characteristic motion and potential for movement that finds its base in WATER. In order for FIRE to complete its radiant transformation, it must be fed adequately by the rising energy of TREE. This energetic cycle is not, then, a series of unrelated phenomena, but a continuum of change, looping back on itself in an endless drama of materialization and diffusion.

In Far Eastern medicine, the various organ systems and functions of the body are seen to be animated, with varying degrees of influence, by this cycle of transformation. Each stage of transformation has biological, emotional and spiritual qualities animated by this energetic transformation. If the various stages of transformation are allowed to complete themselves, an individual's capacity for maintaining a healthy existence is enhanced. If, however, the energies are blocked or stagnated, or if any particular phase becomes overly excited, the effect of the energies becomes perverse, producing disharmony, tension or confusion.

The Five Tastes

The purpose of the seasonal eating program is to help individuals experience the benefits of increased balance and health in life. There are five tastes that are naturally contained in all foods. In TCM, each taste is correlated with a season, a type of warming or cooling energy, and a specific body organ or system. Theoretically, each taste nourishes a specific organ or organ system.

Practically speaking, the more you consciously include a variety of the five tastes in food preparation, the more satisfying and nutritionally enhanced your meals will be. Sometimes just a small amount of a "taste" (e.g. a sprig or two of bitter-tasting parsley leaf) can contribute significantly.

The five tastes are: bitter, salty, sweet, sour and pungent. A food will never contain one exclusive taste; there will always be a variety of tastes. The TCM medical organ connections for each of the five tastes are:

✿ **Bitter** – associated with the early and mid-summer season (FIRE), bitter foods are thought to stimulate the heart and small intestine.

✿ **Salty** – associated with the winter season (WATER), salty foods impart strength and are thought to influence the kidneys and bladder. These foods have a cooling effect and help retain water when the season is dry.

✿ **Sweet** – associated with the late summer season (SOIL), sweet foods are thought to influence the pancreas, spleen and stomach – organs of sugar absorption and distribution. Their nourishing effect is centering and relaxing. The sweet taste refers to natural wholefoods and not the excessively refined sweetness we know from white sugar. Sweet foods include whole grains and vegetables and make up the largest percentage of our meals.

✿ **Sour** – associated with the spring season (TREE), sour tasting foods have a constrictive effect, giving quickening energy. They are thought to influence the liver and gall bladder.

✿ **Pungent** – associated with the autumn season (METAL), the pungent taste in foods gives off a hot, dispersing energy and is said to be beneficial to the lungs and colon. However, an excess of these foods can irritate the intestines. Pungent foods have been known to stimulate blood circulation and, according to traditional Chinese folk medicine, have a natural ability to help break down accumulation in the body. In most culinary cuisines, they are commonly combined with animal protein and with foods high in fat.

It is said that a little of a particular taste can strengthen an organ system, whereas excess can weaken it. Hence, too much sugar weakens our SOIL energy, affecting the stomach, spleen and pancreas, and contributes to digestive problems.

How Foods Fit the Five Tastes

For convenient referencing, the following lists some basic foods that fall into each category of taste.

Bitter – kale, collard greens, mustard greens, parsley leaves, endive, celery, arugula, grain beverages, dandelion, burdock root, sesame seeds, cereal grain coffee substitute, some types of corn

Salty – sea salt, tamari, miso, sea vegetables, sesame salt, umeboshi salt plum, natural brine pickles, soy sauce

Sweet – corn, cooked onions, squashes, yams, cooked grains, cooked cabbage, carrots, parsnips, fruits, sweet potato

Sour – lemon, lime, sauerkraut, umeboshi plum, fermented dishes, pickles, sourdough bread, vinegar, wheat

Pungent – ginger, garlic, raw onions, white radish, red radish, scallions, wasabi, spices, daikon radish (or dried daikon), peppers, horseradish

While most of your meals will contain a minimum of 60% sweet foods (whole grains, vegetables, beans and fruit), you should aim for a full range of other tastes with major meals. The other tastes can be represented in side dishes, sauces and condiments, emphasizing a particular taste you may crave. There is a definite art to meal balancing. The combination possibilities using disease-fighting nutrients are plentiful. The underlying principle dictates that these flavors, while seeming antagonistic (not compatible), are actually, by virtue of meal balancing, complementary.

Meals that include the five tastes will prove much more satisfying, in terms of limiting cravings, and more fortifying. Many of the recipe suggestions I will give you in the following chapters take this into account. An example of this balance factor can be seen in recipes that call for oil; pungent or sour flavors taken in combination with oil help make oils easier to digest. Other examples might be mustard (pungent) with oil, or tamari (salty) with fish, or salt added to water-fried (or sautéed) onions. Eventually, this will become a natural practice as you develop your cooking efficiency and planning ability, and comfortably ease into your new way of eating.

For thousands of years people ate the foods produced in their local environment. People in temperate zones ate the foods of temperate zones – whole grains, beans, fresh seasonal vegetables and fruits, and other products of their regional agriculture. This traditional practice underscores an important principle of macrobiotic eating: *to eat foods that come from the climate zone in which one lives.* Eating foods from the same climate zone makes it easier to come into harmony with our immediate environment.

For example, traditionally, the Eskimo and other people in the far north based their diets around fish and other animal foods found in the Arctic region. Vegetable foods were scarce and a diet high in animal products helped them make balance with their harsh climate, since animal foods generate plenty of heat in the body. Following this principle, people in tropical regions lived on the unique plant and animal species found there. In India, for example, people intuitively adopted a vegetarian or semi-vegetarian way of eating, because minimizing the intake of animal food made it easier to adapt to a hot climate.

Chapter 6

BLOOMING IN SPRING

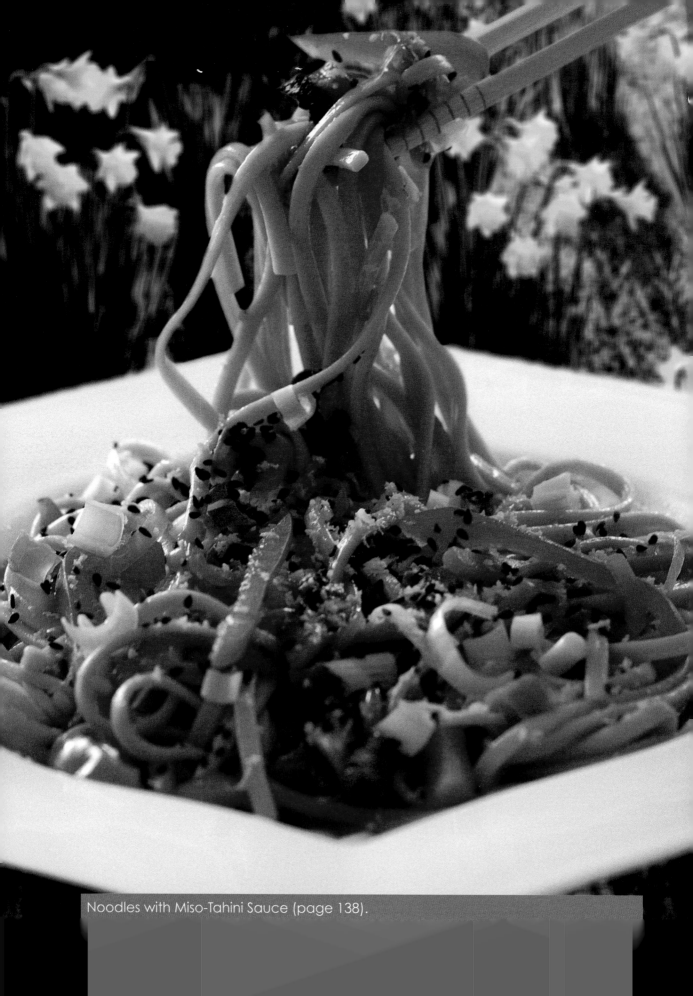

Noodles with Miso-Tahini Sauce (page 138).

Spring for me is the most beautiful time of year. I adore watching the beautiful snowdrops peep through in early February. There used to be many lovely gardens on my walk to school, and I am sure the neighbors did not begrudge me a few wee snowdrops to press into my schoolbooks. Then the crocuses would shoot up with the most beautiful vibrant yellows, purples, and white and blues that filled my world with color.

When you are a child, everything seems so big and awesome, and for me the daffodils around Easter time were the crème de la crème. Big, beautiful, bright heads of sunshine blowing in the wind in various shades of yellow, sitting below the incredible beauty of the apple blossom trees that lined the streets and avenues in shades of white and pink, would tell us that summer was just around the corner.

Spring is such a wonderful time of year, with new buds on the trees and shrubs, and everything coming alive again from the dormancy and hibernation of winter when it seems like the world is asleep. Well, nature has been asleep, resting, but then comes back in full force to fill our lives with color. How clever, what a life plan, what a creation.

General Considerations

Did you ever wonder why we say such things as "put more spring in your step" and "spring into action"? We don't say put more *winter* in your step. Spring is the time when the earth comes alive; light rains and more sun bring life to the surface. Spring is the time of rebirth – the time for opening the windows and cleaning the house. The dietary rules for spring are like house cleaning. This is when the relative lack of activity and heavier eating of the winter months need cleaning out.

Spring is the time of year when the liver and gall bladder present themselves for an annual service. The flavor most often associated with this season is the sour taste, and the relevant vegetables are fresh new-growth greens. These are foods that are seen to promote a gentle cleansing of the liver. Yes, this is the time of year when your body really wants to detox naturally.

Spring is the best time of year to lose weight and lighten the energy of the body. Nature shows us what is needed. It is the use of the new sprouts of greens and foods which release fats and relax the body that is most beneficial. Since winter foods are more likely to have more fats and protein, the use of raw foods and sprouts, along with a lighter approach to cooking, allows the body to release stagnation. As the weather turns sunny, this is a good time to get outdoors and hike, walk and play.

Spending time outside is important. We all need to feel that release of energy that spring represents. As you increase your exercise you will find that your body releases tension and that stretching comes easier. Power walking is a great way to give your metabolism a boost and help remove any winter pounds you may have gathered round the middle during the months that the kidneys required protection from the cold.

Spring is a good time to let go of poor nutritional habits that we might have let get out of hand in the winter months when we were seeking warming comfort. Sometimes the cold winter months create a craving for greater quantities of comfort foods in the diet. This is especially true if you eat dairy food, meat or even oily fish. Spring is also a good time to cut down on food volume. In many cultures you will find that times of fasting take place in the spring. Spring is the time for renewal – time to clean the house.

> *A teaspoon of lemon juice or a few drops of ginger juice added to your water in the morning for a week or two is a good digestive aid to kick off the spring-cleaning. Introducing more sour and fermented foods in your cooking, such as lemon juice, good-quality vinegars and garnishes with a mild hot taste (e.g. scallions or radish), is helpful.*

Quick pickles as a side dish can also help relax that overused liver. In the Recipes for Spring section you will find some great recipe ideas for quick pickle dishes that are quick and simple to make at home. In Chinese medicine the liver is associated with anger and irritability. Try to avoid arguments and make a policy of associating with friends who you can have fun with. Anger causes stress in the body and can lead to stored tension. If you find yourself in an irritating situation, try to get outdoors as soon as possible and go for a good walk.

Something Like Spring

The spring menu is aimed at lightening the load and bringing about flexibility. It is also designed to relax the liver and help to discharge fats and salts from the system. Anyone who has eaten a diet heavy in meats and fats may greatly benefit from following the spring guidelines at any time of year until they feel that their body has found a new and healthy balance.

You may have noticed that "detox" programs have become very popular; most of these use a springtime approach. They use raw foods and often wheat or barley grasses, and they frequently include sour foods such as vinegars to stimulate the liver to discharge fats. The problem is that this kind of approach is often very extreme and exhausting for the body. Simply incorporating sensible spring energy into the daily diet and eating well on a daily basis will produce better long-term results. By all means use spring energy when you need it, but focus more on this strategy when the actual season arrives.

Special Drinks and Home Remedies

Green Juices

Drinks made from the juice of a variety of green vegetables have a rejuvenating effect on the body because they are rich in chlorophyll (the life blood of the plant). They help to purify the blood, build red blood cells, detoxify the body and provide fast energy. Easy to absorb and filled with antioxidants, green juice is the perfect fuel for your body and a great drink in the spring. The juice is easily assimilated as it has a high water content and contains the whole vegetable except for the fiber, which is the indigestible part of the plant. Green juice therefore provides all the healthful ingredients in a form that is easy to digest. Because the micronutrients are broken down, it is easy to absorb and is wonderful for people with digestive issues.

Green-Juice Rejuvenator

Drink your greens – your daily vitamin and mineral cocktail. Here is just one option – feel free to experiment with your own ideas.

1 carrot

1 cucumber

4 celery stalks

1 fennel stalk

Some spinach leaves, kale, chard, or other fresh greens

Tiny piece of ginger root

Parsley sprig

Handful of alfalfa sprouts (optional)

Put all the ingredients through a juicer and add the alfalfa sprouts before drinking. You could also add one teaspoon of a superfood green powder – I use barley grass.

Liver Cleansers

These two drinks are great for helping the liver release the fats stored during the winter and help in any weight-loss program. You can use a cup of these teas once or twice a day, preferably between meals. You may notice that your urine has a strong smell or changes color when drinking these teas – don't be alarmed.

Daikon, Shitake and Kombu Drink

1 dried shitake mushroom

½ cup dried daikon

2½ cm (1 inch) strip kombu seaweed

3 cups spring water

Place the shitake, dried daikon and kombu in a small bowl, rinse and then cover with some water. Leave to soak for about 10 minutes. Discard the soaking water. Slice the shitake and place the ingredients into a pan. Add the spring water, cover and bring to a boil on a medium flame. Reduce the heat and simmer for about 15–20 minutes. Remove and discard the ingredients. Drink the tea while hot.

Note: You can also add half a cup of leafy green vegetables, such as kale, cabbage or watercress. Add the chopped leafy greens at the end and simmer for a further 2 to 3 minutes.

Dried Daikon Drink

Good for removing fat from the cells and reducing excess yang in the body. This is a great tea for the spring to clean the liver after the heavier diet of winter.

1 tbsp dried daikon

1 cup water

Pinch of salt or dash of shoyu

Soak daikon for 10 minutes and remove water if it is too dark. Place daikon, salt (or shoyu) and water in a pan and boil for 5 minutes. Drain and serve.

Recipes for Spring

(Each recipe yields 4 servings)

As with all recipes, you can use these dishes at any time, but they are best in the spring and give you an idea about the kind of cooking and ingredients used. I suggest (even encourage) you to experiment with these and make them your own.

You will see that some of these dishes require more time than others. I wanted to give you an idea of how to make truly tasty treats for you and your friends and family. When in a hurry you can simply refer to the quick meal ideas in Chapter 11.

Soups

Dashi Stock

Dashi stock is an essential ingredient in macrobiotic dishes and Japanese cuisine. It is an earthy-flavored stock made from kombu soaking water and a great base for soups, stews, sauces, noodle broths and dips. Usually dashi is seasoned to taste with a generous serving of shoyu. Often mirin is also added, plus a little juice squeezed from a piece of grated ginger root. This simple soup stock can be stored in the refrigerator and kept for several days. With additional vegetables it can be used as a clear broth served hot or cold.

2 pieces kombu (18 cm/ 5 inches)

3 dried shitake or maitake mushrooms

8 cups water

For a basic dashi, soak the kombu and mushrooms in the water for at least 15 minutes. Remove the mushrooms and thinly slice the caps. Discard the roots, as they can be bitter tasting. Return mushrooms to the water, bring to the boil and simmer gently for 10 minutes. Remove the kombu and keep it to use for cooking, as a condiment or with beans.

Celery Soup

1 onion, finely chopped

4 large sticks celery, peeled and finely chopped

1 large carrot, finely chopped

4 cups Dashi Stock (see page 69)

3–4 sprigs fresh thyme

1 bay leaf

Freshly grated nutmeg

Salt and pepper (optional)

Celery leaves for garnish

Heat the oil in a large saucepan over a medium-low heat. Add the onion and cook for 3–4 minutes, stirring frequently, until just softened. Add the celery and carrot and continue cooking for 3–4 minutes. Season lightly with salt and pepper if desired. Add the stock, thyme and bay leaf and bring to the boil. Reduce the heat, cover and simmer gently for about 25 minutes, stirring occasionally, until the vegetables are very tender.

Allow the soup to cool slightly and remove the thyme and bay leaf. Using a hand blender, purée until smooth. Ladle into warm bowls and garnish with celery leaves and ground nutmeg.

No Cream of Broccoli Soup

2 tbsp olive oil

1 large onion, finely sliced

2 stalks celery, thinly sliced

2 large heads of broccoli florets

4 cups Dashi Stock (see page 69)

Kuzu

Soy milk

Flaked almonds

Sea salt

Heat the oil in a large soup pot and add the onion and celery and a pinch of sea salt. Sauté for 3 or 4 minutes then add the broccoli. Pour the Dashi Stock over the ingredients, bring to a boil and simmer for 20 minutes.

Purée the soup using a hand blender. Mix one heaping teaspoon of kuzu in a little water and add the mixture to the soup along with a generous dash of soy milk. Heat a few more minutes then serve, topped with flaked almonds.

Spring Miso Soup

At the arrival of the spring equinox, it's good to change the ingredients in the miso soup that we eat daily. As spring is the time for the regeneration and cleansing of the liver, the ingredients listed here are magnificent for doing the job. Remember, shorter cooking times for this time of year are also best. This is a great soup to boost the immune system, but do not boil the miso or you will destroy the enzymes.

1 onion, cubed

2 cups butternut squash or pumpkin, cubed

6 cups (or more if desired) spring or filtered water

2 dried shitake or maitake mushrooms, soaked 10 minutes then diced

12 cm (5 inch) piece of kombu or wakame

1 cup dried daikon, soaked for 10 minutes (discard the water)

1 tsp miso per cup of soup

Scallions, finely diced, for garnish

Place onion and butternut squash (or pumpkin) in a pan, cover with one cup of water and bring to a boil. Soak the seaweed for 5 minutes then cut into thin slices and add to the other vegetables. Add the rest of the water and vegetables to the pan, bring back to a boil and simmer for 10 minutes. Whisk miso with a little of the broth and then add to the soup and simmer for 3 minutes. Serve hot, garnished with finely chopped scallions.

Dried Daikon Soup

½ cup dried daikon

3–4 shitake or maitake mushrooms

2 onions

4 cups water

Shoyu

Chopped parsley

Soak daikon and mushrooms for 20 minutes, discard the water and finely dice both vegetables. Cut onions into small pieces and bring to a boil in a pot with a small amount of the water and simmer for 5 minutes. Add daikon and mushrooms and the rest of the water and cook for 20 minutes. Season with shoyu and continue to simmer for 5 more minutes. Serve warm with chopped parsley.

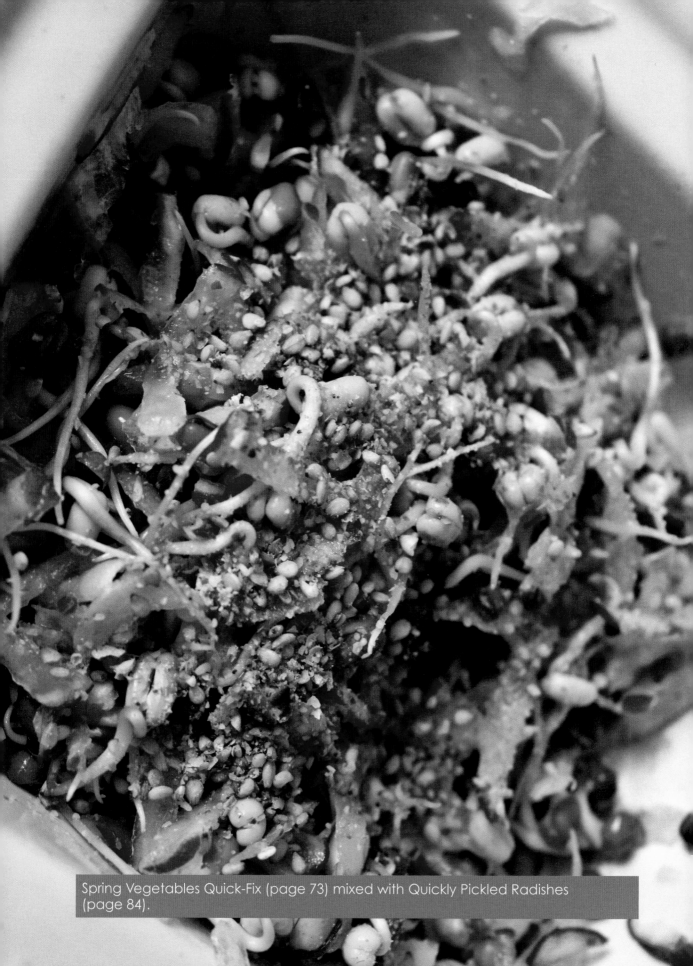

Spring Vegetables Quick-Fix (page 73) mixed with Quickly Pickled Radishes (page 84).

Vegetable Dishes

Greens with Vinaigrette

Lightly cooked greens are full of vibrant color and concentrated goodness. The simple dressing in this recipe complements the slightly bitter flavor of the greens. Carrots and sesame seeds add a great contrast of color and texture.

1 large bunch of leafy greens, e.g. kale or spring greens

1 medium carrot, cut into thin julienne strips

1 tbsp toasted sesame oil

1 tbsp brown rice vinegar

1 tbsp shoyu

1 tbsp toasted sesame seeds

Wash the greens and remove any tough stems or damaged bits from the leaves. Fill a large saucepan halfway with water and bring to the boil. Put as many whole leaves as will comfortably fit into your steamer or colander, and steam over the boiling water until just tender, about 7 minutes. When the greens are tender, immediately remove them from the steamer or colander and plunge into a bowl of cold water to stop the cooking and hold the color. Drain, gently squeeze out excess water, and thinly slice. Cook any remaining leaves in the same way. Steam the carrots for 2–3 minutes, remove, and cool under running water. Drain and set aside.

In a small bowl, whisk together the oil, vinegar and shoyu with a fork. Toss the greens and carrots in a mixing bowl with the dressing. Serve sprinkled with the sesame seeds.

Spring Vegetables Quick-Fix

4 cups cut bok choy

4 cups zucchini, sliced

2 cups bean sprouts

3 tbsp sesame or olive oil

1 tsp ground black pepper

Flaxseed oil

Toasted sesame seeds

Sauté bok choy in oil till the greens darken then add the zucchini till the centers turn slightly translucent. Add bean sprouts and pepper and cook for an additional 5 minutes. Drizzle with some flaxseed oil and sprinkle toasted sesame seeds on top.

Watercress with Tangy Tangerine Dressing

This is a great quick dish for spring; the bitter greens are an aid to weight loss. To keep the dressing on the sweet side, you need more tangerine juice than lemon juice.

1 bunch fresh watercress, rinsed well and hand shredded

¼ cup pecan halves, lightly pan toasted

Juice of 3 tangerines

Juice of 1 lemon

Pinch of sea salt

Pinch of black pepper

Generous dash of brown rice vinegar

¼ cup extra virgin olive oil

Place shredded watercress in a medium salad bowl and add pecans. Make the dressing by whisking together all the remaining ingredients until combined (you can make enough for several meals and put in the refrigerator for later). Chill watercress and dressing separately, tossing together just before serving.

Any Steamed Greens

Greens are great simply steamed for a few minutes. Wash the greens and cut them in narrow strips to cook quicker and release the flavor. Put them in a steamer, bring the water to a boil and place the steamer inside and cover. Most greens will be tender within 3 to 5 minutes. If you want to jazz them up, pour a little oil and good vinegar over them or drizzle with any of the sauces you find in this book.

Spring/Collard Greens with Citrus Dressing

Greens are full of vitamins and nutrients, and delicious when served as a simple side dish.

8-10 large spring/collard green leaves, washed and drained well

Juice of ½ orange

1 tsp umeboshi paste

Cut the middle stem from each of the leaves and chop the stem finely or discard if tough. Slice the greens finely. Bring half an inch of water to a boil in a shallow saucepan. Place the greens and stems (if using) in the water and cook for 2 to 3 minutes. In a small bowl, mix the orange juice and umeboshi paste with about one tablespoon of water to make the citrus dressing.

When the greens are tender, remove them from the pan and drain. Place in a serving bowl and drizzle with the dressing. Lightly toss and serve.

Steamed Vegetables

This is a good dish to move stagnant energy around your liver and lungs.

1 bunch watercress

1 cup bok choy

1 large carrot

4 radishes, halved

1 tbsp shoyu

1 tbsp brown rice vinegar

Place vegetables in a steamer basket and steam over boiling water for 2 minutes. Transfer to a serving dish and sprinkle with the shoyu and brown rice vinegar.

Grain Dishes

Grain Burgers

2 cups leftover (cooked) millet or rice

1 onion, finely grated

½ carrot, finely grated

1 tbsp chopped parsley

1 tsp each thyme, marjoram

Pinch of dried sage

½ tsp sweet paprika

¼ tsp turmeric

Pinch of black pepper

Salt and shoyu to taste

Wholewheat flour

Sunflower frying oil

Mustard to serve

Mash grain in a large bowl along with the onion and carrot, then add the parsley, herbs, sage, spices, salt, pepper and shoyu. Adjust seasoning to taste. Wet your hands and form the mixture into burger shapes, then roll them in wholewheat flour and fry until golden brown. Serve with Double Cranberry Chutney (see page 212).

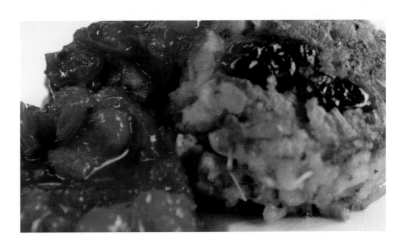

Polenta with Shitake

1 tbsp olive oil

1 clove garlic, minced

1 cup diced shitake mushrooms

4 cups spring water

½ tsp sea salt

1 cup polenta

2 tbsp minced fresh basil

Place the oil in a pan, add the garlic and shitake and lightly sauté. Add the water and sea salt and bring to a boil. Drizzle the polenta into the broth and stir. Cook covered on a low flame for about 15 minutes, stirring now and again to stop it from sticking. Add the basil and mix.

Spring Quinoa Salad with Zesty Lemon Dressing

2 cups water

1 cup quinoa, washed and drained

1 jar organic corn

¼ cup chopped scallions

1 cup chopped walnuts

1 cup chopped cucumber

1 apple, peeled and chopped

¼ cup chopped mint leaves

2 tbsp chopped fresh cilantro

2 tbsp chopped fresh mint

2 tbsp chopped fresh parsley

¼ cup pitted black or green olives

Sea salt

Bring the water and a pinch of salt to a boil in a large saucepan. Add the quinoa and bring the water back to a boil. Cover the pan and reduce the heat to low so that the contents simmer until all the liquid has been absorbed. This usually takes 20–25 minutes. Remove the pan from the heat and allow the quinoa to cool.

Transfer the quinoa to a large mixing bowl and add the remaining ingredients. Mix well. Drizzle Zesty Lemon Dressing (see page 77) over the salad and stir in. Season the salad with a pinch of sea salt. Allow the salad to sit for 30 minutes to allow the flavors to develop before serving.

Zesty Lemon Dressing

¼ cup freshly squeezed
lemon juice

¼ cup extra virgin olive oil

Zest of ¼ lemon

Mix the lemon juice and olive oil, and stir in the lemon zest. Serve over Spring Quinoa Salad (see page 76).

Asian Style Millet

Millet is one of the natural wonders of the culinary world and a versatile grain with a delicious nutty flavor. It cooks up creamy and stew-like, or you can pan roast it to make it fluffy and light, enhancing and supporting the other flavors in a dish, as in this elegant, exotic grain dish. Millet can also be used to make fantastic-tasting tabbouleh.

1 cup millet, rinsed well

3 cups filtered water

2 tsp toasted
sesame oil

4 slices fresh ginger, finely
minced

2 cloves fresh garlic, finely
minced

1 carrot, finely diced

1 sweet potato, finely
diced (parboiled before
sautéing)

1 large onion, cut into
diagonal slices

1 tsp fresh ginger juice

1 tbsp brown rice syrup

1 tbsp brown rice vinegar

Handful of pistachios or
nuts of your choice

Soy sauce

Heat a deep, dry pan over medium heat. Drain millet well before toasting so that it toasts evenly and does not burn. Add to pan and toast until millet puffs and begins to pop – about 5 minutes. Add water and a sprinkle of soy sauce and bring to a boil. Reduce heat, cover and simmer for about 30 minutes, until the liquid is nearly absorbed. Remove from heat, cover and allow to stand for 10 minutes. Fluff up with a fork and transfer to a serving bowl.

At the same time as the millet is cooking, heat another pan with the sesame oil over a medium flame. Add minced ginger and garlic and cook for 2–3 minutes. Add carrot, sweet potato and onion and cook until tender. Sprinkle with a little soy sauce and stir in ginger juice and rice syrup. Remove from heat and stir in brown rice vinegar and nuts. Fold into the hot millet and serve warm, as millet tends to stiffen as it cools.

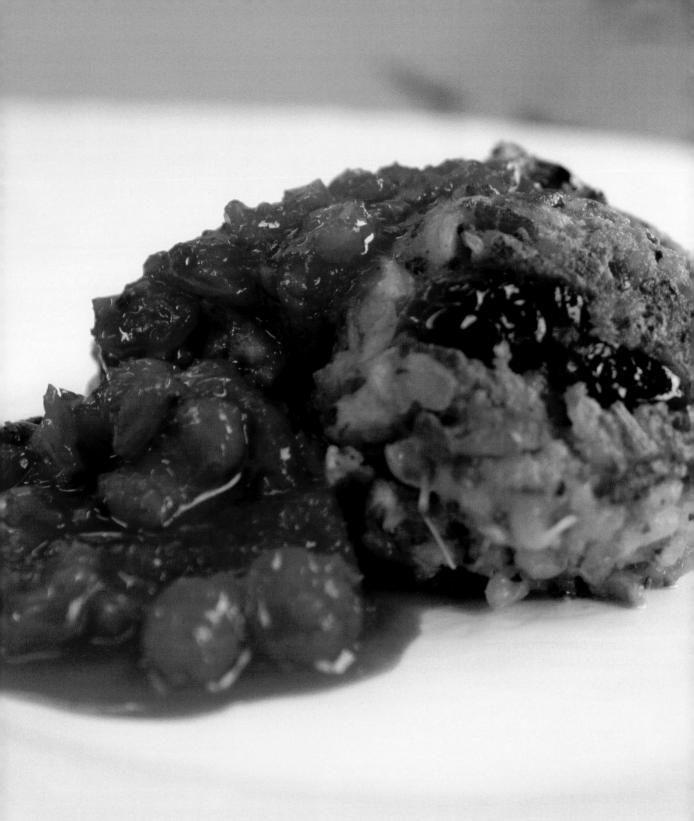

Grain Burgers (page 75) with Double Cranberry Chutney (page 212).

Beans and Bean Products

Marinated Tofu Steaks

Steaks

1 pack tofu, cut into 8 equal slices

3 tbsp rice flour

Sesame oil

marinate

1 clove garlic, crushed

2 small scallions, diced

4 tbsp mirin

4 tbsp shoyu

1 tbsp toasted sesame seeds

Dipping Sauce

1 tbsp shoyu

1 tbsp juice from freshly grated ginger

1 tbsp grated daikon

Mix the marinade ingredients in a bowl and marinate the tofu for 30 minutes.

Place the dipping sauce ingredients in a small bowl and mix. Serve in a small bowl to share.

Remove the tofu steaks from the marinade and dust with the flour. Heat the sesame oil in a wok or pan and fry the tofu for 2–3 minutes on each side until golden brown.

Serve with wholegrain brown rice and steamed vegetables.

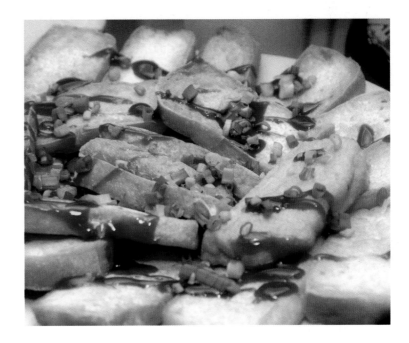

Tempeh Bolognese

This classic Italian pasta sauce is made with crumbled tempeh instead of ground meat. Try it over udon noodles, spaghetti, polenta or puréed cauliflower.

1 tbsp + 1½ tsp olive oil, divided

1 medium onion, peeled and finely chopped (1½ cups)

1 large carrot, finely chopped (½ cup)

1 cup finely chopped celery

1 tsp dried oregano

3 cloves garlic, minced (1 tbsp)

1 pack tempeh

1 tbsp shoyu or tamari

½ cup water

1 can organic diced tomatoes

½ cup dry white wine or sake

2 tbsp organic tomato paste

¼ cup tahini

Heat one tablespoon of oil in a large pan over medium-high heat. Add onion, carrot, celery, oregano and garlic. Cook, stirring often, for 5–6 minutes or until vegetables are browned. Meanwhile, heat remaining one and a half teaspoons of oil in separate pan over medium heat. Add tempeh and brown for 2 minutes on each side. Add soy sauce (shoyu or tamari) and half a cup of water. Cook the tempeh for 5 minutes more, or until all the liquid has been absorbed. Crumble tempeh into small pieces with spatula. Stir the tempeh, tomatoes, wine (or sake), and tomato paste into onion mixture. Reduce heat to medium-low and simmer, partially covered, for 10 minutes. Stir in tahini and simmer for 5 minutes more. Add some water if you prefer a thinner consistency. Add additional shoyu or tamari to taste.

Greek-Style Lentil Burgers

½ cup dried green lentils

1½ cups filtered water

2 tbsp olive oil

1 small onion, chopped (1 cup)

½ red bell pepper, diced (½ cup)

4 cloves garlic, minced (4 tsp)

1 can chickpeas, rinsed and drained

1 cup loosely packed parsley leaves

½ cup pitted Kalamata olives

½ pack tofu

2 tsp ground cumin

1 tsp ground coriander

1 tsp salt

½ tsp ground black pepper (optional)

1 cup plain breadcrumbs

¾ cup finely grated carrots

½ tsp baking powder

Cook the lentils in twice the quantity of water for 35 minutes or until the lentils are soft to the bite. Drain. Heat the oil in a pan over medium heat. Add onion and bell pepper, and sauté for 7 minutes. Stir in garlic. Blend chickpeas, parsley, olives, tofu, cumin, coriander, salt and pepper in food processor for 2 minutes, or until smooth. Stir chickpea mixture, breadcrumbs, carrots and baking powder into lentils, along with the sauté from the pan. Shape into eight patties. Layer patties between parchment paper and freeze for 15 minutes. Preheat grill to high. Brush frozen patties with oil and cook for 6 minutes on each side. Burgers served with Pickled Beets puréed to a sauce (page 119).

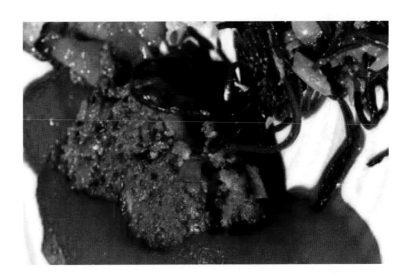

Sauces, Salads and Side Dishes

Crunchy Boiled Salad with Pumpkin Seed Dressing

¼ cup carrots, cut into diagonals

1 cup green beans

¼ cup red radishes, cut into quarters

1 cup broccoli florets

1 tbsp fresh parsley

Place five centimeters (two inches) of water in a medium pan and bring to a boil. Place the carrots in a steamer basket and steam in the boiling water for 2 to 3 minutes. Remove and place in a mixing bowl. Repeat these steps with the green beans, radishes and broccoli, individually. Add the parsley to the vegetables.

Drizzle Pumpkin Seed Dressing (see below) over the vegetables, toss lightly and serve.

Pumpkin Seed Dressing

1 tbsp pumpkin seeds

1 tbsp shoyu or tamari

1 tbsp water

1 tbsp grated fresh ginger

1 tbsp freshly squeezed lemon juice

Toast the pumpkin seeds in a small pan over medium heat until brown.

Combine the shoyu (or tamari) and water in a small saucepan and simmer over low heat for 3 minutes. Remove the pan from the heat, add the ginger, lemon juice and pumpkin seeds and stir well.

Arame with Onions and Toasted Walnuts

Like all other seaweeds, arame strengthens and nourishes the blood.

2 onions, finely sliced

Olive oil

Pinch of sea salt

1 cup arame, rinsed and soaked in cold water for 15 minutes

½ cup water

Soy sauce

Apple juice concentrate

Lemon rind, finely grated

Toasted walnuts for garnish

Sauté the onions with some olive oil and a pinch of sea salt for 15 minutes uncovered, until they are translucent and have a rich aroma. Drain the arame and add to the onions, together with half a cup of water. Cover and simmer gently until all the water has been absorbed – approximately 20 minutes. Season to taste with some soy sauce (shoyu or tamari), apple juice concentrate and lemon rind. Garnish with toasted walnuts.

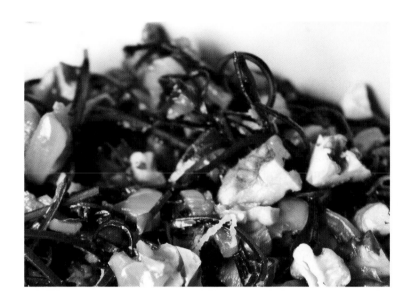

Coleslaw

½ white cabbage, chopped

1 large carrot, chopped

Handful scallions, chopped

⅓ cup walnut oil

⅓ cup brown rice vinegar

1 tsp mustard

1 cup soy mayonnaise

Juice from olives or pickles

Pinch of sea salt

Mix the cabbage, carrots and scallions in a large salad bowl. (A food processor may be used for quickness.) In a separate bowl, mix the walnut oil, brown rice vinegar, olive or pickle juice, sea salt and mustard with the soy mayonnaise. Add to the mixture. Allow the dressing mixture to stand for at least an hour.

Pour the dressing over the cabbage, carrots and scallions and mix in well. Can be eaten immediately or will keep in the refrigerator for 4 to 5 days.

Quickly Pickled Radishes

A spring tonic for replenishing and cleansing the body.

1 bunch radishes, sliced

2 tbsp umeboshi vinegar

1 cup water

Place the radish slices in a bowl. Add the vinegar to one cup of water in a small pan and bring to a boil. Remove from the heat and pour the liquid over the radishes. Store for up to 5 days in the refrigerator.

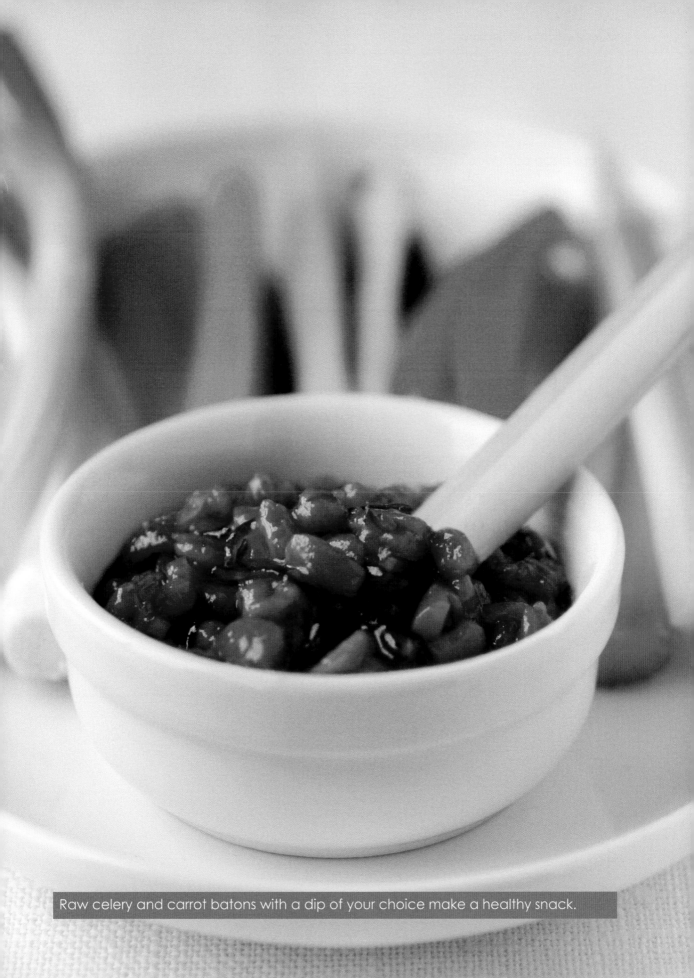

Raw celery and carrot batons with a dip of your choice make a healthy snack.

Pressed Salad

3 cups napa cabbage, cut into 2½ cm (1 inch) strips

½ cup daikon, cut into matchsticks

½ cup seedless cucumber, cut into matchsticks

½ cup carrot, cut into matchsticks

2 tsp sea salt

Mix all the vegetables and salt in a bowl. Put the mixture into a pickle press and allow to sit for at least 30 minutes.

Remove from the press and gently squeeze the vegetables to remove excess liquid. Return to the bowl.

Sweet Mustard Sauce

1 tsp shoyu

2 tsp Dijon mustard

1½ tbsp maple syrup

Combine all ingredients in a bowl and mix well. Pour over the pressed salad. You can make larger quantities and store in the refrigerator in a glass dish. Have a small portion with lunch or dinner.

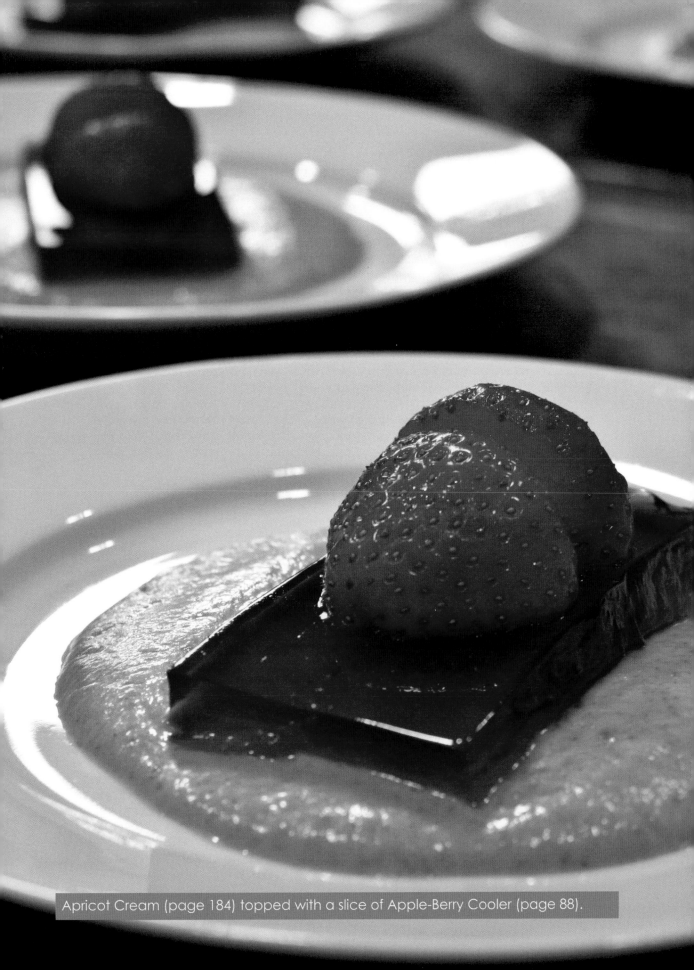

Apricot Cream (page 184) topped with a slice of Apple-Berry Cooler (page 88).

Desserts

Agar-Agar (Kanten)

Agar-agar is made from seaweed and used as a gelling agent in place of gelatine in jellies. Agar-agar's natural gelling ability, mild flavor and total lack of calories have made it a favorite with health-conscious and vegetarian cooks around the world. Even at room temperature, it sets quickly as it cools, and seals in the natural flavor and sweetness of any fruits and vegetables used, as well as having the benefit of a naturally high-fiber content. Agar-agar is a vegetable gelatine, which appeals to vegans because true gelatine is generally made from calves' feet.

Light and refreshingly cool, agar-agar dishes are especially popular in the spring and summer, but the gelling agent can be used with vegetables and stock to make beautiful molded aspics any time of the year.

You can test each recipe by taking a spoonful of the heated mixture and dropping it onto a cold plate. If the mixture doesn't set in a few minutes, sprinkle a few more agar-agar flakes into the pot and continue to simmer for a few more minutes.

Apple-Berry Cooler

1½ liters (2½ pints) organic apple or apple-strawberry juice

1–2 rounded tbsp agar-agar flakes

1 basket (250 g) of fresh berries (e.g. raspberries, strawberries), whole or sliced

Small pinch of sea salt

Pour the juice into a small saucepan and add the salt. Sprinkle the agar-agar flakes on top, bring to a gentle simmer, and gently stir it now and then with a wooden spoon. Simmer for 3 minutes and then remove from the heat. Pour over the whole or sliced berries in a mold or a bowl. When it's cooled down a bit, put the bowl in the refrigerator – it'll be firm in about 1–2 hours. Then either scoop out or turn out the whole jelly by gently pulling the sides of the jelly away from the mold or bowl and inverting the dish over a plate.

Note: Soft fruits such as berries, cherries, peaches and melons do not need to be cooked with agar-agar. However, firmer fruits such as apples and pears need to be peeled, chopped and cooked in the agar-agar and juice mixture to soften them.

Alternatively allow to cool in a flat dish and cut into squares.

See photograph on page 121.

Lemon Pudding

2 cups apple juice

2 cups rice milk

Juice and zest of 1 lemon

4 heaping tbsp agar-agar flakes

2 heaping tsp kuzu or arrowroot powder

1 tsp vanilla essence

⅓ cup rice malt syrup

Pinch of salt

Bring apple juice, rice milk, lemon zest, salt and agar-agar to the boil in a saucepan. Simmer for 5 minutes until the agar-agar flakes have dissolved. Make a paste with the kuzu or arrowroot with two teaspoons of water and add to the pan, stirring constantly. Simmer for 5 minutes. Stir in vanilla essence, lemon juice and rice syrup. Remove from heat, transfer to a dish and leave to cool until set – approximately 1–2 hours.

Blend in a food processor until smooth, and serve.

Toasted Seed Bars

1 cup pumpkin seeds

1 cup sunflower seeds

1 cup sesame seeds

1 cup pine nuts

½ cup rice syrup

In a large pan or wok, toast the seeds until crisp and popping, or alternatively place them on a baking sheet and roast in the oven. Warm the rice syrup in a small pan, then pour over the seed mixture and mix thoroughly until consolidated.

Place on a baking sheet and pat down evenly. Leave to cool and then cut into bite-size pieces.

Chapter 7

FIT AS A FIDDLE FOR SUMMER

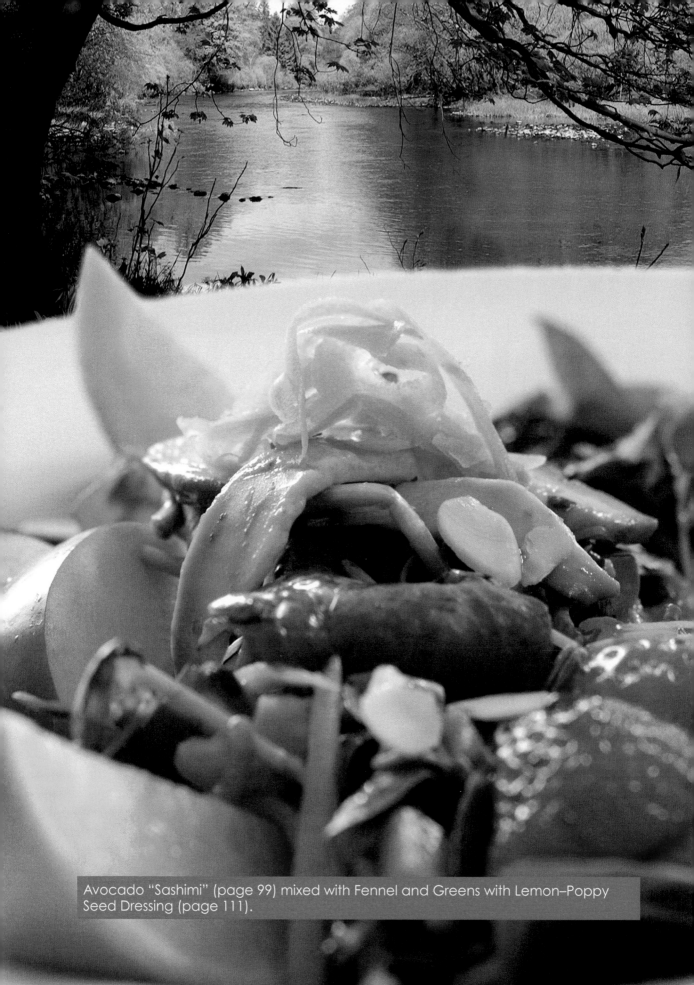

Avocado "Sashimi" (page 99) mixed with Fennel and Greens with Lemon–Poppy Seed Dressing (page 111).

"Summertime, and the livin' is easy." You may remember these words from the song "Summertime," all about lazy days when everything seems to slow down. Summer is a good time to forget our worries and let our hair down. As children, we use to play outside all day in the warmth of the sun during the summer school holidays. Yes! Scotland does have sunshine – it doesn't rain all the time, I promise you.

The flowers were in full bloom, the perfume from rose bushes wafted in the air, the hanging baskets overflowed with an abundance of colors bobbing about in the breeze; when playing in the sun, everyone seemed happier than at any other time of the year. This makes sense to me now that I understand more about the seasons. Summer is the season of high energy, joy and passion. It is when nature is at its full and glorious height.

When I was twelve I worked in the local fruit shop during the school holidays and adored merchandising and dressing the shelves with all the wonderful colors and shapes of the fruits and vegetables. Not many children of my age would have been excited about that exactly, but I was happy. I would rise early, around 6 am, and go to the fruit market with my boss to make the daily purchases. Everything was grown locally, everything was fresh, and everything was chemical free and packed with nutrition. Sorting through the grains and beans, even at that young age, made me happy – I adored all of that. So even though I was unaware at that time where my love of nature and the seasons would take me in forty years' time, I had definitely started my training and journey towards studying natural health care.

General Considerations

Summer is a time of openness and peace ... and the living is easy. The excitement of spring gives way to flowering and ripening of life. Summer is a time to let troubles drift away and enjoy life. A time to stop and smell the flowers.

This is the time of the greatest expansion of energy in the cycle; it is the most abundant time for growth. The foods that are most needed when the weather is warm are salads, fruits and green vegetables – and lighter cooking is required. Cooking needs to be subtle as well, so be sure not to overcook. This kind of food will help us to keep our cool, but if we use any animal food in our diet, the amount needs to be reduced or, better still, eliminated.

The energy of summer nourishes the heart and the small intestines. It provides us with a good opportunity to lighten the diet, cut down on salty foods, eat more raw foods, enjoy fruits and generally relax the system. Sunny days and warmer weather call out for an orderly and relaxed way of being. This is a great time to get rid of the stress in your life; practice lying on the grass and watch the clouds like you did as a child.

You will find that this is the easiest time to cut the sugar, coffee, black tea or alcohol out of your diet. It is usually a good idea to increase the amount of pure water you drink (always at room temperature). When you rise in the morning, hydrate your cells with water. We lose approximately half a cup of water each night when we sleep, and the cells need hydrating when we awake. Remember that the brain is composed of 80% water so you will feel more alert when you give the body what it needs. You might also try dry skin brushing before having a shower (it's wonderful) – it will not only make your skin velvety smooth but also increase circulation, creating a healthy glow.

Something Like Summer

Diseases of the heart are provoked by eating too much meat and dairy food, causing the blood to thicken and the arteries to become clogged with excess fats. The light and simple foods of summer may be helpful for anyone having these problems at any time of year. Simplicity is the key – nothing fancy or complex. Raw vegetables and lightly cooked dishes help restore the balance and calm the system.

The healthy diet of summer uses less oil and oily foods and concentrates on the abundant variety of vegetables available. Foods that overheat the body are not good for the heart and therefore avoided, and salt is usually reduced. Use the summer approach when you want to do the heart a favor.

If you are a smoker and want to quit, drink some Dandelion Root Tea (see recipe on page 95) and chew on a little bitter dandelion root when you crave a cigarette – it helps suppress the urge.

Special Drinks and Home Remedies

Heart Tonic Drink

Prepare a special drink consisting of daikon greens and other hard leafy greens (two parts), dried shitake mushroom (one part), corn (one part), cabbage (one part), and wakame or nori (one part). Add four to five times as much water. Bring to a boil and simmer for 15 minutes. Drink one cup daily for 3 weeks.

Dandelion Root Tea

This tea is helpful in lowering high blood pressure. Use dried dandelion root, available from most natural food stores and herbal shops. Place one teaspoon of the dried leaves in a teapot with boiling water. Leave to infuse for 5 minutes. You can reuse the tea by adding additional boiling water to the teapot for a second cup.

Daikon and Carrot Drink

This is the best combination of ingredients to make a powerful tea that will kick-start your weight-loss program. Spicy and pungent, this tea is designed to help dissolve hardened fat deposits that have accumulated deep within various organs, inhibiting their function. The drink works to dissolve fat, while adding minerals to create strong blood quality.

1 tbsp grated carrot

2 tbsp grated daikon (or if using dried daikon, soak for 10 minutes in water then discard the water)

1 cup water

Dash of shoyu

½ sheet toasted sushi nori, shredded

1 umeboshi plum, pitted and diced

Place carrot and daikon in a pan with the water and shoyu, bring to a boil and simmer for 4 or 5 minutes. Stir in shredded nori and umeboshi plum, and simmer for a few more minutes.

Recipes for Summer

(Each recipe yields 4 servings)

It is wise to resist the habit of drinking cold beverages, because they cool you off for a short period of time but then you get hot again. If you do drink them, sip them slowly and you will find you are more comfortable. Eat soft fruits and berries to cool down. Introduce couscous, bulgur wheat or quinoa into your salads and add fresh corn to your diet.

Soups

Carrot and Almond Soup

2 tbsp olive oil

1 onion, finely chopped

1 leek, thinly sliced

4 carrots, thinly sliced

6 cups Dashi Stock (see page 69)

½ cup flaked almonds

1 tbsp fresh lemon juice

Snipped fresh chives for garnish

Heat the oil in a large saucepan over a medium heat and add the onion and leek. Cover and cook for about 3 minutes, stirring occasionally, until just softened. Do not allow them to brown. Add the carrots and Dashi Stock. Bring to the boil and then simmer gently for 45 minutes until the vegetables are tender. Purée with a hand blender, adding the flaked almonds halfway through blending, and continue to blend until you have a nutty-looking texture. Add the lemon juice and serve with the snipped chives. Delicious.

Wakame White Miso Summer Soup

The golden color and light, sweet flavor of this nutritious soup makes it a delightful choice during the warmer months.

15 cm (6 inch) piece of wakame

6 cups Dashi Stock (see page 69)

1 large carrot, thinly sliced

6 small scallions, cut into 1 cm (½ inch) pieces

4 heaping tsp sweet white miso

Soak the wakame for 10 minutes. Cut away any tough ribs and slice the fronds into 2 cm (1 inch) pieces. While it's soaking, bring the Dashi Stock to the boil, add the carrot and simmer for 10 minutes. Then add the scallions and simmer for a few more minutes. Add the wakame to the soup, simmer for 2 more minutes, and then remove from the heat. In a cup, thin the miso with a little bit of the hot soup, and then add this liquid back into the pan. Stir the miso in well, and leave the soup for a few minutes before serving, so that the flavors can mingle.

White Bean–Vegetable Soup

4 pieces kombu (postage-stamp size)

4 cups spring water

½ cup dried white beans (soaked overnight and drained) or other cooked organic beans

½ cup diced onion

¼ cup white mushrooms, including stems, sliced into thin strips

¼ cup diced celery

White miso, sea salt and black pepper (optional) to taste

Flat-leaf parsley for garnish

Soak the kombu in one-quarter cup of spring water for 30 minutes. Place the beans in a pressure cooker with the kombu and 2 cups of water plus the soaking water. Cover and bring up to pressure. Cook for 45 minutes, remove from heat and allow the pressure to come down on its own.

In a pot, layer bottom to top as follows: onion, mushrooms, celery and cooked white beans. Add 1½ cups water or more to cover the ingredients and bring to a boil over medium heat. Reduce heat to low and simmer for 20 minutes.

Season to taste with white miso, salt and black pepper. Transfer to bowls and garnish with parsley.

Vegetable Dishes

Steamed Greens

Wash and slice the greens – watercress, bok choy, Swiss chard, collards or other greens. Place the vegetables in a stainless-steel steamer in a pot with two centimeters (one inch) of boiling water, cover and steam for 2–3 minutes, depending on the texture of the vegetables you are using (they should be a bright green color and crispy). Wait until the water is fully boiling before you put in the vegetables. You can sprinkle a little brown rice vinegar, umeboshi vinegar or shoyu over them when serving. Eat while warm as a side dish or for breakfast when following a weight-loss program.

Watercress with Parsley

Watercress is packed full of vitamins and nutrients and is a perfect bitter side dish. It is an excellent dish for a weight-loss program.

3 bunches watercress, chopped

½ cup parsley, finely chopped

¼ tsp tamari

In a shallow saucepan, bring one centimeter (half inch) of water to a boil. Add the watercress and cook for 3 minutes. Add parsley and tamari. Cook the greens for 2 minutes. Drain and serve.

Walnut Celery Sticks

¼ cup walnuts

1 tbsp orange juice

½ tsp orange rind

1 tsp brown miso

5 celery stalks

Roast the walnuts in a dry pan until toasted – about 5 to 8 minutes. Remove from the pan and finely chop. Place the orange juice, orange rind and miso into a small bowl and mix well. Add the walnuts and mix together. Place a small amount of the mixture along the center of the celery. Cut into bite-size pieces and serve.

Kale falls into three groups: true kale, Siberian kale and collards. True kale (Scotch kale, curly-leaved kale, or borecole) usually has dark green or glaucous leaves with heavily frilled margins. Few greens can match the nutritive power of kale – it is an excellent source of fiber, folate, vitamins A, C and E, calcium, potassium, iron, riboflavin and sodium.

Kale and Broccoli Stir-Fry

This is a great recipe for a quick lunchtime stir-fry and uses kale (or dark-leafed cabbage greens or spinach) and broccoli.

1 tbsp vegetable oil

2 cloves garlic, peeled and crushed

10 fresh shitake mushrooms, washed and chopped

½ block tofu (optional), small diced

1 head of broccoli, chopped into medium-sized chunks

1 head curly kale, washed, stalk removed, and thinly sliced

1 tbsp sesame seeds

3 tbsp tamari

1 tsp barley miso paste

Heat the oil in a wok until hot, add the garlic and the mushrooms, stir well and cook for 5 minutes until the mushrooms are lightly browned and their juice has evaporated. Add the diced tofu (if using) and cook on a high heat for 3 minutes, stirring until it starts to brown. Add the broccoli, stir and cover, and cook for 5 minutes or until it turns bright green. Add the kale, cover and cook for 2 minutes until it starts to wilt. Remove the wok from the heat. Stir in the seeds with the tamari and miso paste, mixing well.

Avocado "Sashimi"

1 medium-sized ripe avocado

Juice of 1 lemon

2 tbsp shoyu

¼ cup spring water

1½ tsp wasabi powder (optional)

Halve the avocado lengthwise, slicing through to the pit. Twist halves and pull apart. Remove the pit and then peel the avocado. Thinly slice the avocado halves lengthwise and coat with the lemon juice to stop them going brown. Mix the shoyu and water, dividing the mixture into individual dip saucers – allow one tablespoon per serving.

Add one drop of water at a time to the wasabi powder and mix until it forms a thick paste. Place a small dollop of wasabi on each plate of avocado "sashimi" for guests to mix into their shoyu dip.

To eat, pick up each avocado slice with chopsticks, dip into the shoyu and wasabi, and enjoy alongside nori rolls.

Grated Daikon Salad

To add a little color to your table, try this lively salad.

5 cups torn greens

1 cup peeled, shredded daikon

1 cup endive leaves

½ cup shredded beet

½ cup toasted, shelled pumpkin seeds

⅓ cup sunflower sprouts

2 tsp lime juice or lemon juice

2 tsp dried basil

1 tsp rice syrup

1 tsp dried thyme

8 red radishes, sliced

Black sesame seeds

Place all ingredients in a large bowl, toss well and sprinkle with black sesame seeds.

Grain Dishes

Macro Paella

1 tsp saffron threads

2 tbsp olive oil

2 cloves garlic, finely diced

1 onion, finely chopped

2 tomatoes, finely chopped

1 red pepper, finely chopped

1 yellow pepper, finely chopped

1 green pepper, finely chopped

Fresh green beans, finely chopped

2 artichokes, peeled and sliced, or a handful of asparagus (whichever is in season)

1 pack tempeh, seitan or tofu

1 organic vegetable bouillon cube, mixed in 1 liter (1¾ pints) of water

Tamari

1 cup paella rice

Lemon wedges

Soak the saffron threads in a bowl of water and set to one side. In a large paella pan, heat the olive oil and add the garlic, onion and tomatoes, and sauté until soft. Add the peppers, green beans and artichokes, and cover with the bouillon stock. Add the tamari and leave to simmer on a low heat for 30 minutes or more, until the vegetables are al dente (firm to the bite), adding more water if necessary. Add the rice and the saffron soaking water and simmer for 25 minutes, covering with foil for the last 10 minutes. Add more water if necessary. Serve with lemon wedges arranged around the pan.

Unless you can find the perfect paella rice, the best rice that I have found to use in this dish is Uncle Ben's wholegrain brown rice, as it is not glutinous but lighter and absorbs the saffron well.

Chilled Soba Noodle Salad

1 pack soba noodles

2 tsp toasted sesame oil

½ cup watercress

½ cup red lettuce leaves

2 scallions, finely chopped

1 tbsp toasted pumpkin seeds

1 sheet nori, finely shredded

Dash of shoyu

Dash of brown rice vinegar

Dash of toasted sesame oil

Bring a large saucepan of water to a rapid boil and add the soba noodles. Stir to ensure all the noodles are separated. Cook 8–10 minutes then rinse in cold water to stop cooking. Stir in the toasted sesame oil and set aside. Put the noodles in a large mixing bowl, mix with the salad leaves and drizzle with some shoyu, brown rice vinegar and a little more toasted sesame oil. Sprinkle with toasted pumpkin seeds, top with the scallions and shredded nori, and serve.

Bulgur with Pine Nuts and Raisins

1 cup bulgur

2 cups water

½ cup pine nuts

1 onion

1 tsp olive oil

½ cup raisins

Scant pinch of cinnamon

Make the bulgur in the usual manner by adding two cups of water to a pan, bring to a boil, add the bulgur and reduce to a simmer for 20 minutes. Toast the pine nuts in a dry pan. Sauté the onion in the olive oil and after 3 or 4 minutes, add the pine nuts and raisins, mix and cook for a few minutes. Stir into the bulgur and sprinkle some cinnamon on top.

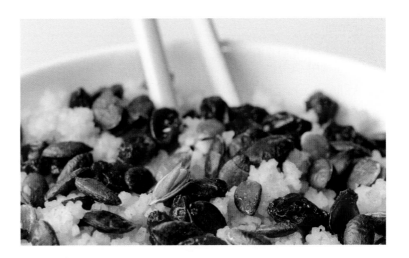

Couscous with Carrot Juice

1½ cups organic carrot juice

1 cup couscous

1 red onion, finely diced

1 tbsp umeboshi paste

Pinch of sea salt

Bring the carrot juice to a gentle boil in a saucepan, add in the couscous and the pinch of sea salt, stir and then turn off the flame. Cover and let it sit for 5 minutes until all the juice has been absorbed. Mix the onion with the umeboshi paste and add to the couscous.

Brown Rice, Vegetable and Tofu Stir-Fry with Sliced Almonds

A quick, easy and delicious dish that can be made with any vegetables.

1 tbsp extra virgin olive oil

4 medium carrots, julienned

1 cup chopped fresh shitake mushrooms

2 stalks celery, julienned

1 tsp minced fresh ginger

2 cloves fresh garlic, thinly sliced

2 small zucchini, julienned

1 large white or yellow onion, cut on the diagonal

1 red onion, cut on the diagonal

1 brick of tofu, cut into 1 cm (½ inch) cubes

1 cup finely chopped leafy greens, such as kale or bok choy

1 cup sliced almonds

3 tbsp tamari

½ cup water

2 cups cooked brown rice

Pinch of sea salt

In a large wok, heat the olive oil until it's very hot but not smoking. Add the carrots, mushrooms, celery, ginger, garlic and a pinch of salt and stir fry over medium-high heat for 5 minutes. Add the zucchini, onions and tofu and cook for 5 minutes more. Add the greens and stir fry until they are just wilted (add a little water if necessary). Stir the almonds into the mixture. Mix the tamari with one-third of a cup of water, pour over the stir-fried vegetables and cook for another 5 minutes.

Transfer the vegetables to a serving dish and serve with cooked brown rice.

Veggie Nut Bulgur Salad

1 cup water

½ cup bulgur

½ onion, diced

½ carrot, diced

½ cup celery, diced

¼ cup walnuts, chopped in small pieces

¼ cup pine nuts

1 tsp sesame seeds

Tamari

1 tsp parsley

¼ cup sauerkraut with juice

Pinch of sea salt

Bring the water to a boil, add the bulgur and the salt, cover the pan and reduce heat to low. Simmer for about 15 minutes until the bulgur is soft and fluffy. Place the bulgur in a large mixing bowl and stir to cool it off. Toast the pine nuts in a small pan over medium-low heat for 5–7 minutes until they are golden brown. Toast the sesame seeds in a small pan over medium-low heat for 3–5 minutes until they start to pop. Add a few drops of tamari after 3 minutes and stir. When the bulgur is cool, add the vegetables, nuts, seeds, parsley and sauerkraut with juice, and mix thoroughly.

Beans and Bean Products

Deep-Fried Crumbled Tempeh and Onion Salad

Organic sunflower oil

1 pack tempeh (crumbled)

1 clove garlic, crushed

1 onion, diced

Mixture of salad greens

1 carrot, grated

Toasted sesame seeds

Chopped parsley for garnish

Heat the oil in a deep pan and deep fry the tempeh until it becomes crisp and golden. Sauté the garlic and onion together in a saucepan for 5 minutes until translucent and then mix together with the deep-fried tempeh in a bowl. Prepare a mixture of greens, such as fresh arugula and crisp fresh lettuce, and mix in the tempeh and onions.

Serve with one of the delicious sauces or salad dressings on pages 117–118. Dress with the grated carrot, sprinkle with toasted sesame seeds and garnish with chopped parsley.

Agedashi Tofu

A taste of vegan zen.

2 blocks of silken tofu

Organic sunflower oil for deep frying

4 tbsp rice flour

2 tsp grated fresh ginger root for garnish

1 scallion, finely sliced on the diagonal, for garnish

Dashi Broth

1¼ cups Dashi Stock (see page 69)

4 tbsp shoyu

4 tbsp mirin

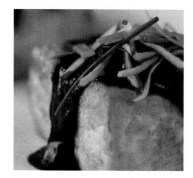

Drain the tofu on paper towels until dry, changing the paper towel as required. Place all the ingredients for the dashi broth in a saucepan and bring to a gentle boil. Heat the oil to about 180°C/350°F in a heavy-based deep-frying pan. Cut each tofu block in half and then half again. Dust with the flour then gently slide the tofu into the oil and deep fry until crisp and golden. (*Note*: Don't dust the tofu with the flour until you are ready to fry it; otherwise it will become sticky.)

Arrange the tofu in bowls and ladle some dashi broth to one side of the tofu. Garnish with the grated ginger and scallion.

Peanut Seitan

This makes a delicious lunch and can be served in a pita, garnished with fresh salad greens. Alternatively, serve it with a noodle salad.

1 tsp toasted sesame oil

1 pack seitan, drained and cut into ½ cm (¼ inch) slices

2 tsp tamari

1 tsp mustard

½ cup water

2 cups fresh greens

3 tbsp roasted organic peanuts

1 cup bean sprouts (optional)

Add the oil to a large pan and sauté the seitan slices in the oil over medium heat for about 4 minutes. Dissolve the tamari and mustard in the water and pour the mixture over the seitan. Add the greens and peanuts, cover and simmer over medium heat for 5 minutes. Turn off the heat and mix in the sprouts, if using (the heat from the other ingredients will cook the sprouts). Serve either with noodles or in a pita.

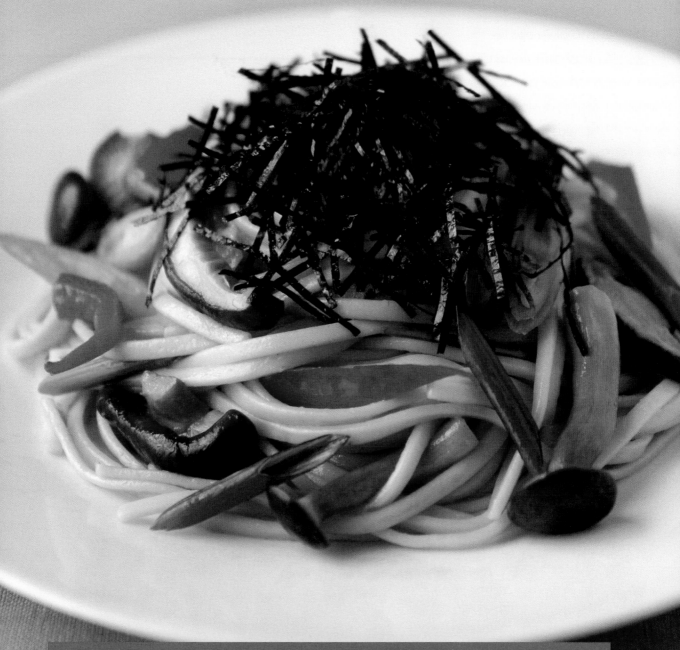

Mushroom Soba Noodles Topped with Shredded Nori (page 172).

Summer White Bean Salad

2 cans white beans, drained

3 cloves garlic, minced

1 red onion, minced

½ cup chopped fresh parsley

2 tbsp olive oil

2 large tomatoes, diced

⅓ cup sliced black olives

1 tbsp red wine vinegar

1 tsp lemon juice

Salt and pepper to taste

Over a low heat, combine the beans, garlic, onion and parsley in olive oil. Heat for just one minute, or until fragrant. Remove from the heat and mix together with the remaining ingredients. Serve warm, as is, or chill before serving.

Tofu, Asparagus and Red Pepper Stir-Fry over Quinoa (Part 1)

Quinoa

1 cup quinoa

2 cups filtered water

Pinch of sea salt

Quinoa is a delicious, easy-to-cook grain and is very high in protein.

Place the quinoa and water in a saucepan. Add salt, cover and reduce heat to low. Cook until the water has been absorbed and quinoa has opened (as in sprouting) – about 20–25 minutes. Remove from heat.

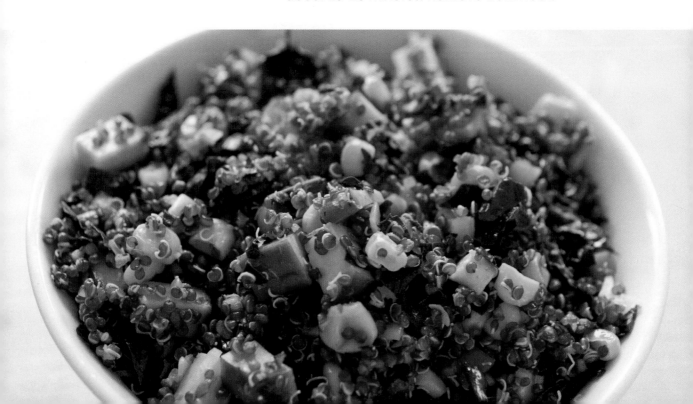

Tofu, Asparagus and Red Pepper Stir-Fry over Quinoa (Part 2)

1 tbsp extra virgin olive oil

3 cloves fresh garlic, finely diced

3 tbsp fresh ginger, cut into fine matchstick pieces

1 red onion, sliced into thin half moons

2 tbsp red peppers (from natural foods store – they come sliced in a jar)

1 block tofu, cut into 2½ cm (1 inch) cubes

Bunch of asparagus, tips snapped off and stalks thinly sliced diagonally

Grated zest of 1 orange

2 tbsp freshly squeezed lemon juice

Shoyu

While the quinoa is cooking, heat the oil in a pan or wok over a medium heat. Add garlic, ginger, onion and a splash of soy sauce, and sauté until the onion is tender and translucent – about 4 minutes. Stir in the red peppers (thinly sliced) and a splash of soy sauce and sauté for a few minutes. Add tofu on top of the vegetables but do not stir in, season with one tablespoon of soy sauce, cover and reduce the heat to low and simmer until the tofu is cooked through – about 8 minutes. Add the asparagus and orange zest and a splash of soy sauce. Cover and cook until the asparagus is bright green – about 5 minutes. Remove from the heat and gently stir in the lemon juice.

Arrange the quinoa in a shallow bowl and spoon the stir-fry over the top. Delicious!

Sauces, Salads and Side Dishes

Cucumber Salsa

2 baby cucumbers, deseeded and finely sliced into ribbons

12 red radishes, sliced into fine ribbons

1 pinch of sea salt

1 tbsp brown rice vinegar

1 tbsp rice mirin

Mix together the cucumbers, radishes and salt in a small mixing bowl and top with the vinegar and mirin.

Tabbouleh

Be creative and adjust the ingredients to fit the number you are serving, or make enough to last for the next day's lunch. Make it up – make it fun.

Bulgur

Olive oil

Garlic, minced

Onion, diced

Zucchini, diced

Tamari

Mirin

Olives, green and black, sliced

Cucumber, diced

Chickpeas

Corn

Sweet rice vinegar

Parsley

Toasted pumpkin seeds

Toasted sunflower seeds

Pan roast the bulgur in a dry pan and then add twice the amount of liquid and simmer on a low heat until the water has been absorbed. Transfer to a large serving bowl and fluff up with a fork. Heat a pan with the olive oil and sauté the garlic, onion and zucchini in a little tamari and mirin until soft to the bite. Let cool and add to the bulgur. Mix the olives, cucumber, chickpeas and corn into the bulgur. Drizzle with olive oil and vinegar, and garnish with parsley, pumpkin and sunflower seeds.

Wakame with Grated Apple

Few strips of wakame

Spring water

Juice of 1 orange

Zest of 1 orange

1 apple, peeled and grated

Soak a few strips of wakame for about 10 minutes in spring water. Drain and cut into small pieces and remove any ribbed pieces. Add some orange juice and zest to the wakame. Top with grated apple and serve.

Guacamole

This quick and easy recipe makes a delicious spread for toast and crackers, or a dip for sticks of celery and cucumber. Use soft ripe avocados – the skin should peel easily and the flesh should be easy to mash.

1 large or 2 small ripe avocados, peeled and pitted

¼ small onion, grated

1 tbsp umeboshi plum vinegar

Juice of ¼ lemon

Sprig of parsley, finely chopped

Mash the avocados with a fork. Add all the other ingredients and mix well with the fork. Serve with hot pita bread and olives.

Sweet Potato Salad with Apple and Avocado

More a meal than a side dish, this potato salad gets its protein from avocado and pumpkin seeds, both good sources of essential fatty acids. Nutrient-rich corn and diced apple give it crunch. Try serving it over a bed of spinach or arugula.

2 large sweet potatoes, peeled and cut into 1 cm (½ inch) cubes

1 cup frozen corn

¼ cup unsalted pumpkin seeds

1 medium red apple, diced (1 cup)

½ scallion, finely chopped (½ cup)

¼ cup chopped cilantro

¼ cup lime juice

2 tbsp olive oil

½ avocado, finely diced

Place sweet potatoes in large saucepan and cover with water. Bring to a boil and cook for 3 minutes. Add corn and cook for 1 to 2 minutes more, or until the potatoes are tender. Drain in a colander and rinse under cold water to cool. Drain well. Toast pumpkin seeds in a dry pan over a medium-high heat for 3 to 4 minutes, or until the seeds begin to pop. Transfer to a plate and cool. Combine apple, scallion, cilantro and lime juice in a large bowl. Stir in sweet potatoes, corn and oil, and season with salt and pepper, if desired. Stir in avocado and toasted pumpkin seeds just before serving.

Dulse Salad with Watercress

This is rich in minerals and good for strengthening the blood.

15 cm (6 inch) dulse strip

2 tbsp pumpkin seeds

1 tbsp olive oil

1 bunch watercress, washed and cut into small lengths

1 tbsp shoyu

Place the dulse in water and leave it to go soft. Toast the pumpkin seeds in a lightly oiled frying pan over a medium heat, stirring frequently to prevent burning. Cut the dulse into similar lengths as the watercress. Pour a small amount of water into the frying pan, heat the water, add the dulse and soften. Then drain the water, add the watercress and sauté for 1 or 2 minutes, stirring occasionally. Turn off the heat, season with shoyu and transfer to a serving bowl. Mix in the pumpkin seeds before serving.

Arugula Salad

1 large bunch arugula

1 tsp umeboshi vinegar

2 tbsp olive oil

Toasted pine nuts

Wash and spin-dry the arugula, then place in a salad bowl. Make the vinaigrette by mixing the olive oil and umeboshi vinegar. Pour over the greens and toss to coat the salad leaves. Top with toasted pine nuts.

Fennel and Greens with Lemon–Poppy Seed Dressing

4 cups mixed salad greens

½ cup fresh herbs – parsley, dill or cilantro

10–12 cherry tomatoes

1 bulb fennel, finely sliced

Sea salt to taste

Place the greens, herbs, tomatoes and fennel in a large serving bowl. Sprinkle with a little sea salt and drizzle with Lemon–Poppy Seed Dressing (see below). Gently toss the salad and serve.

Lemon–Poppy Seed Dressing

2 tbsp white miso

2 tbsp lemon juice

¼ cup water

¼ tsp poppy seeds

Whisk the miso, lemon juice, water and poppy seeds together until blended.

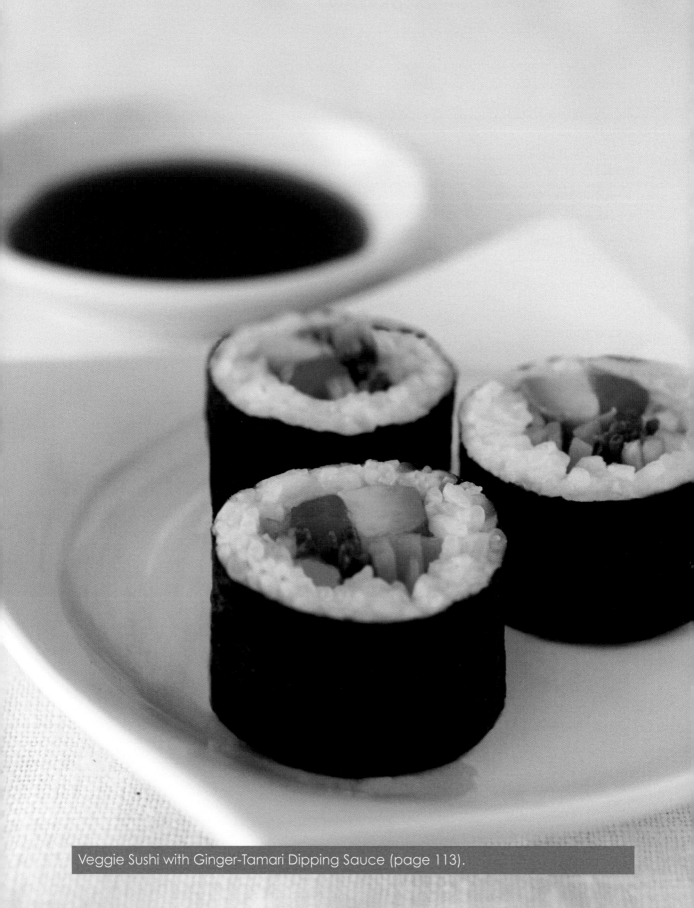

Veggie Sushi with Ginger-Tamari Dipping Sauce (page 113).

Veggie Sushi with Ginger-Tamari Dipping Sauce

As well as an appetizer, sushi makes a wonderful lunch or main course.

1 cup brown sushi rice

1 tbsp brown rice vinegar

½ tbsp mirin

4 sheets toasted nori

1 tbsp black or brown toasted sesame seeds

1 small carrot, cut into strips

¼ cucumber, cut into strips

½ avocado

Handful of watercress

1–2 pieces pickled daikon, cut into thin strips, or sauerkraut

1–2 tsp umeboshi paste or a tiny piece of umeboshi plum (chopped finely)

Cook the rice and allow it to cool to room temperature, or use leftover rice. Place the rice in a large bowl and drizzle it with the brown rice vinegar and mirin, then gently toss the rice.

Lay a nori sheet, shiny side down, on the sushi mat. Spread a quarter of a cup of rice over the nori using the rice paddle or your hands dipped in water, leaving a quarter of the nori bare on the top edge. Sprinkle a quarter of the sesame seeds over the rice. Make a canal with the rice paddle or wooden spoon across the middle of the rice-covered nori sheet. Place some carrot, cucumber, avocado, watercress and daikon or sauerkraut in neat lines across the canal. Add a thin line of umeboshi paste across the vegetables. (*Note:* You may spread some peanut butter along the vegetables or try making your own fillings.) Starting with the end nearest to you, roll the sushi, making sure the filling is contained in the middle of the roll. Unroll the mat, moisten the top edge of the sheet, and roll until the nori is sealed.

Cut the sushi into halves, and then quarters, using a slant or straight cut. Dip your knife into a bowl of water mixed with some vinegar after each cut, for easier cutting. Serve with Ginger-Tamari Dipping Sauce (see below).

Ginger-Tamari Dipping Sauce

2 tbsp tamari or shoyu

2 tbsp water

¼ tsp grated fresh ginger

Mix ingredients together and place in individual serving bowls.

Mediterranean Chickpea Platter

Serve with Tabbouleh (see page 108) or a green salad tossed with lemon vinaigrette.

1 tbsp extra virgin olive oil

1 zucchini (about 350 g/12 oz), cubed

2 cloves garlic, minced

¼ tsp salt, divided

2 tbsp tahini

3 tbsp lemon juice

1 tbsp water

1 can chickpeas or cannellini beans (rinse well to remove surface salt)

3 tbsp chopped fresh parsley, plus more for garnish

2 medium tomatoes, sliced

½ medium red onion, thinly sliced

¼ cup crumbled tofu cheese

¼ cup halved, pitted briny black olives, such as Kalamata

4 pieces of wholewheat pita bread, warmed and cut in half or into wedges

Heat the oil in a large nonstick pan over medium heat. Add zucchini, garlic and one-eighth teaspoon salt, and cook, stirring occasionally, until the zucchini is soft and beginning to brown – about 8 minutes. Meanwhile, whisk tahini, lemon juice, water and the remaining one-eighth teaspoon salt in a medium bowl. Stir in the chickpeas (or beans), parsley and the zucchini. Arrange the chickpea-zucchini salad, tomatoes, onion, tofu cheese, olives and pieces of pita bread in lines on a platter. Serve at room temperature or chilled, and sprinkle with more parsley, if desired.

Sweet Red Miso Marinade

½ cup brown rice miso paste

½ cup mirin

½ cup brown rice syrup

2 tbsp sake

Put all the ingredients in a saucepan and bring to a simmer over a medium heat, stirring all the time with a wooden spoon. Reduce the heat to low once the mixture begins to boil. Continue to stir and let the mixture reduce to the consistency of thick yogurt. Leave to cool at room temperature before transferring to a jar – it will keep in the refrigerator for up to 8 weeks. Use to marinate tofu and tempeh.

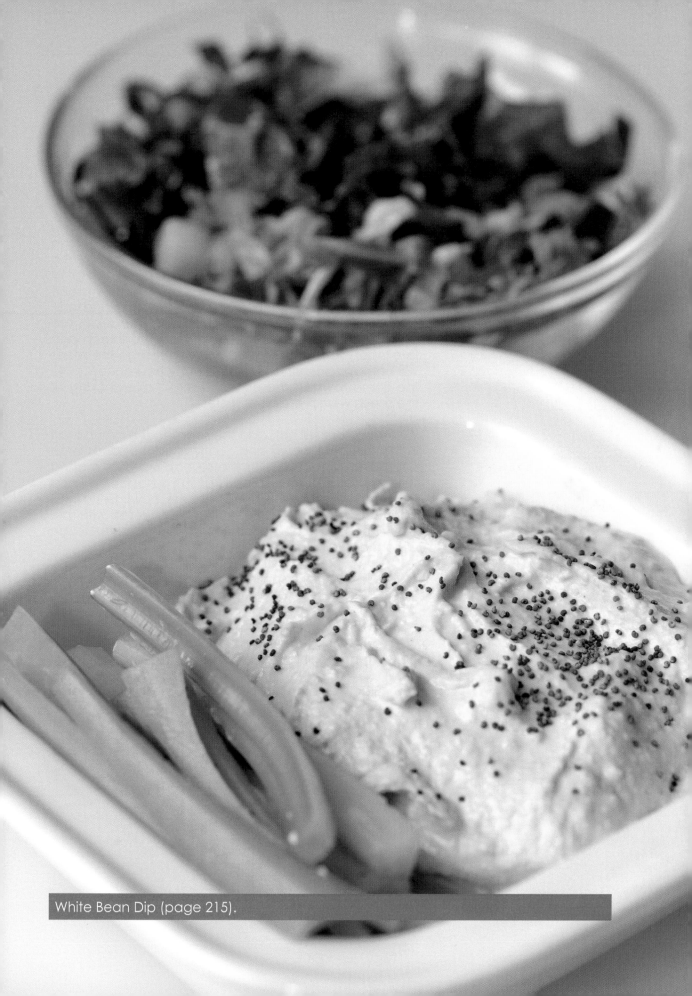

White Bean Dip (page 215).

Gomashio

Gomashio is roasted sesame seeds and sea salt. In addition to its use as a condiment, it is used medicinally to quickly strengthen the blood. It provides an immediate yangizing effect and can help offset extreme yin conditions and reactions.

1 part sea salt

16 to 18 parts sesame seeds

Wash seeds in a fine-mesh strainer and allow them to dry. Dry roast the sea salt in a stainless-steel frying pan over a medium-high flame, until it turns grey. Place the salt in a suribachi (Japanese grinding bowl) or mortar, and grind into a fine powder. Roast the seeds on medium heat and, while roasting, gently push the seeds back and forth with a wooden spoon to avoid burning. The seeds are done when they crush easily between the thumb and forefinger – about 5–10 minutes. At this stage the seeds will begin to pop and give off a nutty fragrance. Lower the flame towards the end and avoid overcooking or the seeds will have a bitter taste.

While they are still hot, add the seeds to the ground salt in the suribachi. Slowly and gently grind the seeds in an even circular motion with the suribachi pestle, making sure to use the grooved sides of the suribachi to grind against, instead of the bottom of the bowl. Grind until each seed is crushed and thoroughly covered with salt. Allow the gomashio to cool and then transfer to an airtight container to serve.

✿ Use gomashio sparingly over grain or vegetables or salad dishes – about one teaspoon per day.

✿ Medicinally, gomashio is helpful for neutralizing acidity in the blood, relieving tiredness, and strengthening the nervous system.

✿ Black sesame seeds can be used in the same way.

Basic Salad Dressing

Handful of parsley

1 cup olive oil

2 tbsp balsamic vinegar

½ tbsp shoyu

Pinch of sea salt

1 tbsp mustard

Lemon juice

Black pepper

Place all the ingredients into a blender and adjust ingredients according to taste. Store in a sealed glass jar in the refrigerator – it will keep for up to 5 days.

Tahini Miso Dressing

Tahini is a thick, smooth paste made from ground sesame seeds. Serve this dressing over cooked or raw vegetables, or as a dip or spread.

2 tbsp light miso

1 tbsp tahini

½ tsp tamari or soy sauce, or a pinch of sea salt

½ tsp lemon juice

Spring water, as needed

Place the light miso, tahini, tamari, lemon juice and water in a blender and blend until smooth and creamy.

Creamy Lemon Ginger Dressing

Use this dressing over a grain dish or cooked and raw vegetable dishes.

110 g (4 oz) soft tofu, cut into cubes

2 tsp ginger juice

3 tbsp fresh lemon juice

3 tbsp extra virgin olive oil

3 tbsp flaxseed oil

2 tbsp spring water

2 tbsp scallions, white parts, finely chopped

1 tsp sea salt

Water and soy sauce mixture

Boil the tofu in a water and soy sauce mixture for about 4 minutes. Place all the ingredients in a food processor and blend until smooth and creamy.

Choose from a variety of dried or fresh garden herbs like parsley, chives, rosemary, sage or thyme, to change the flavor of the dressing. Try using different oils.

To vary the dressings, you can add chopped basil, parsley or chives to the mixture. Or try barley, chickpea or rice miso instead of a light miso.

Orange Ume Dressing

This is a great dressing to serve on green or noodle salads in the summer or over a selection of steamed vegetables or fresh steamed greens.

3 tbsp sesame seeds

Juice of ½ lemon

Juice of 1½ oranges

2 tsp umeboshi purée, or 1 umeboshi plum, chopped (pit removed)

1 tsp finely chopped scallions or chives

2 tbsp sesame or olive oil

Toast the sesame seeds in a dry frying pan over a medium heat for 2–3 minutes, stirring constantly with a wooden spoon. Pour them out of the pan into a blender. Add all the other ingredients into the blender except the scallions or chives, and blend until smooth. Mix the scallions or chives in at the end, and chill for half an hour before serving.

Pickled Beets

3 beets, peeled and sliced

1 small onion, sliced

1 bay leaf

½ cup organic apple juice

½ cup water

2 tbsp shoyu

2 tbsp brown rice vinegar

Place the beets, onion and bay leaf in a pan with the apple juice, water, shoyu and vinegar. Bring to a boil and reduce the heat. Simmer for 10 minutes. The beets will keep for several days refrigerated in a glass jar. Alternatively purée to a cream and serve as a sauce over Grain Burgers (see page 75).

Desserts

Strawberry Mousse

2 cups apple juice

2 cups rice milk

6 tbsp agar-agar flakes

4 tbsp arrowroot powder

½ cup rice syrup

1 basket (250 g) of strawberries, washed and halved

1 tbsp white almond butter (optional)

Pinch of salt

Mint leaves and strawberries for decoration

In a small pot bring to a boil the apple juice and rice milk, adding the salt and agar-agar, stirring occasionally. Simmer for 5 minutes or until the flakes melt. Dissolve the arrowroot in a few tablespoons of cold water, slowly stir it in the boiling mixture and cook for a few minutes. Add the rice syrup and white almond butter, if using. Place the strawberries in a flat baking dish, pour the hot liquid on top and allow to cool. When set, blend until smooth and creamy. Serve decorated with mint leaves and fresh strawberries.

Almond Cream

2 cups almonds

1 cup soy, almond or hazelnut milk

¼ cup rice syrup

2 tsp vanilla extract

Pinch of sea salt

Preheat oven to 160°C/325°F. Place the almonds in a single layer on a sheet pan or cookie tray and bake for 10 minutes. Place soy milk, rice syrup, vanilla and sea salt into a blender. Blend for 10 seconds to mix and add the nuts. Continue blending the mixture until smooth, then chill for 30–45 minutes in the refrigerator. Makes about 2½ cups.

Pecan or Almond Nuggets

4 cups almonds or pecans, pulverized

1 tsp arrowroot powder

½ cup rice syrup

½ cup barley malt

1 tsp vanilla

Desiccated coconut

Mix the almonds or pecans with the arrowroot, and add the rice syrup, barley malt and vanilla. Mix until the nuts and syrup are evenly distributed. Place some water in a bowl and moisten your hands with water to keep the mixture from sticking. Pinch off a piece of the mixture and shape into small balls. Roll in the desiccated coconut. Keep chilled until ready to serve.

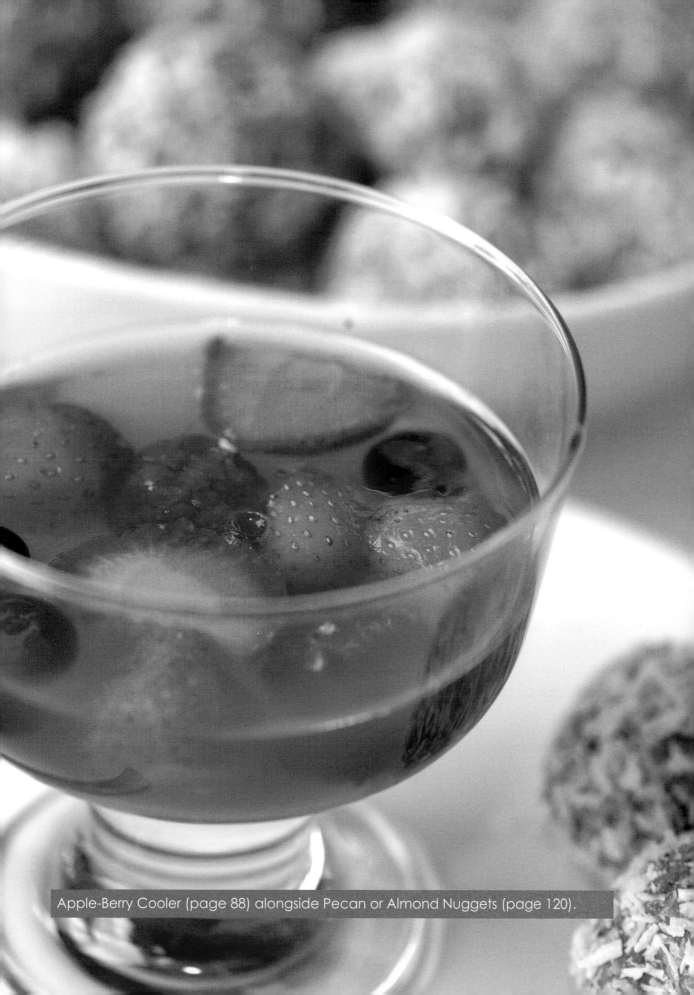

Apple-Berry Cooler (page 88) alongside Pecan or Almond Nuggets (page 120).

Chocolate Tofu Pudding

175 g (6 oz) 100% cacao chocolate, coarsely chopped

1 tbsp vegetable oil

1 block soft tofu, well drained

¼ cup pure maple syrup

¼ cup vanilla or plain soy milk

1 tsp lemon juice

¼ tsp vanilla extract

1 tbsp tahini

1 cup (125 g) fresh strawberries, hulled and sliced, or whole raspberries

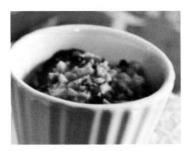

Heat the chocolate and oil in a double boiler over barely simmering water. Whisk until smooth. Remove the bowl from the water and let the chocolate cool for 20 to 30 minutes. Meanwhile, cut the tofu into thick slabs, and place on a triple layer of paper towels. Press firmly on the tofu to squeeze out as much water as possible, changing the paper towels if necessary. Put maple syrup, soy milk, lemon juice, vanilla extract and tahini into a food processor. Crumble the tofu into the mixture and purée until smooth, scraping down the sides with a spatula as necessary. Add the melted chocolate and process until well blended. Transfer the pudding into six custard cups or small bowls. Cover each with plastic wrap and refrigerate for 2 to 3 hours, or until softly set. To serve, top with berries.

Pear Trifle with Cashew Nut Cream

1¼ cups apple juice

1 tbsp agar-agar flakes

1 tbsp lemon juice

4 crunchy organic cookies

Zest of 1 lemon

2 soft sliced pears

1 cup cashew nuts, boiled for 30 minutes, drained and rinsed

½ cup white grape juice

Mint leaves for garnish

Toasted pistachio or walnut pieces for garnish

Rice syrup for drizzling

Black sesame seeds

Heat the apple juice and whisk in the agar-agar and lemon juice. Simmer until the agar-agar flakes dissolve. Crush the cookies, mix with the lemon zest and place in a dessert bowl. Layer the sliced pears over the cookies. Slowly pour the apple juice jelly over the pears and put in the refrigerator to set. Meanwhile, blend the cashew nuts and grape juice, adding the juice slowly until the mixture becomes thick and creamy (use more grape juice if necessary). Pour over the top of the trifle and garnish with mint leaves and toasted pistachio or walnut pieces, and drizzle some rice syrup sparingly. Top the trifle with black sesame seeds and chill in the refrigerator.

Chapter 8

FLOURISHING IN LATE SUMMER

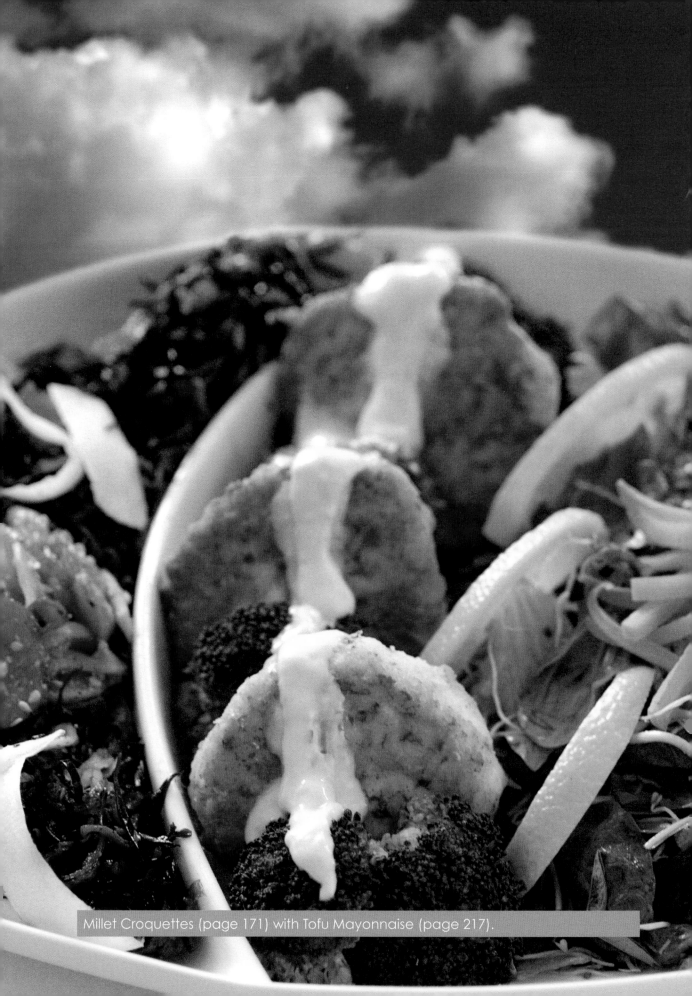

Millet Croquettes (page 171) with Tofu Mayonnaise (page 217).

We don't often hear about late summer as a unique season but this hasn't always been the case. In many countries around the world the transition from summer into autumn was seen as a very specific time of year. It was the time after the harvest and extended through September, but in some places only up until the end of August depending on the local weather. It is that time when the first hints of autumn are present, but the leaves have not yet fallen.

Late summer is a time when "sweet cooking" is recommended. This means that there is more roasting of vegetables so that they caramelize and the sugars are released. The grains for this season are millet and rice. Late fruits, such as pears and apples, are fresh and work well in desserts. White bean dishes and garbanzo beans (chickpeas) are good choices.

In late summer we should be feeling energetic, strong and confident, because rising yin energy has plateaued, relaxed and surrendered to the descending yang energy. It is the time of year when we prepare ourselves for the coming of cooler weather and the winds.

General Considerations

The time of late summer is a time for settling in and achieving balance; the dramatic energies of spring and summer are waning and things are beginning to quiet down. The focus here is on strengthening, stabilizing and getting both feet solidly on the ground.

The physical considerations here are the spleen, the pancreas and the immune system. There may have been a tendency to eat more sugars in the summer in the form of fruits or desserts, so the pancreas needs to be soothed. There may also have been a tendency to drink more and deplete mineral stores. The focus on sweet-tasting foods containing complex sugars takes the stress off the pancreas and calms the system.

Problems with blood sugar can often be improved very simply by adapting a more healthy diet. The biggest culprit is the overconsumption of simple sugars, such as white sugar, fructose, molasses and even honey. Many men and women with type II diabetes have recovered completely by establishing the kind of diet I am suggesting here and getting good exercise daily.

Something Like Late Summer

The energy of late summer is nourishing to the stomach, spleen and pancreas and to the immune system. It is important to bring balance to our eating since it is easy to eat too much sweet food during the high summer. It is a good idea to use the natural sweetness of squash and other sweet vegetables. Baking these vegetables so that they become sweeter is nice as well. The key is complex carbohydrates.

The immune functions and lymphatic system of the body need activity to operate at peak function. Both pancreatic health and problems with the immune system respond very well to increased levels of exercise. This exercise should be vigorous. Seaweeds, especially when eaten in miso soup, are also helpful when the immune system is challenged.

Special Drinks and Home Remedies

Kuzu Drink

Kuzu root starch remedies can be used to treat indigestion, colds and aches and pains. Eating foods made with kuzu have the same effect and it is considered an incredible preventative medicine in Japan and China. Kuzu is fantastic for neutralizing stomach acidity and relaxing tight muscles. With added ginger juice and chopped umeboshi plums, the drink is especially potent and tastes amazing. It is very strengthening for the spleen and immune system.

1 heaping tsp kuzu

1 cup spring or filtered water

1 umeboshi plum, pitted and finely chopped

1 tsp juice squeezed from freshly grated ginger

Dash of shoyu

In a small saucepan, thoroughly dissolve the kuzu in cold water. Add the umeboshi plum and simmer over a medium heat, stirring frequently with a wooden spoon. As soon as the mixture begins to bubble around the edges, stir constantly until the kuzu thickens and becomes translucent. Simmer gently for a couple of minutes and then remove from the heat. Add the freshly grated ginger juice, and shoyu to taste.

Ume-Sho-Bancha Tea

Great for controlling digestion and strengthening the blood and circulation. This is an excellent tea for stomach disorders, lack of appetite, nausea, tiredness and headaches caused by excess yin or anemia.

1 cup hot bancha tea

½ umeboshi plum

½ tsp shoyu

Soak the plum in a small amount of tea, then add the rest of the tea. Add shoyu, stir well and drink.

Sweet Vegetable Tea

This tea is good for relaxing the body and muscles. It is especially beneficial for softening the pancreas and helping to stabilize blood sugar levels. A small cup may be taken daily or every other day in the mid to late afternoon. The tea helps to satisfy the desire for something sweet and reduce cravings for simple sugars and other stronger sweets.

Use equal amounts of four sweet vegetables, finely chopped (e.g. onion, carrot, cabbage and sweet winter squash). Place three to four times as much water in a pan, bring to a boil and add the chopped vegetables. Allow to boil uncovered for up to 3 minutes, then reduce the flame to low, cover and let simmer for 20 minutes. Strain the vegetables from the broth and drink at room temperature.

Apple-Kuzu Drink

This drink is helpful for reducing fever and providing an energy boost to children and adults who are weak and lack energy. In addition, an apple-kuzu drink stimulates the appetite and relieves constipation, as well as de-acidifying and relaxing the intestines. This is a drink that I make for myself when I want to relax.

1 cup apple juice

1 tsp kuzu

Small pinch of sea salt

Heat the apple juice and salt in a small pan over a medium heat until bubbles form at the sides. Dissolve the kuzu in a bit of cold water and add to the apple juice, stirring constantly to avoid lumps forming. Simmer until the kuzu thickens and the color changes from chalky white to translucent. Drink warm.

Recipes for Late Summer

(Each recipe yields 4 servings)

Soups

Millet and Sweet Vegetable Soup

1 cup millet, washed

½ butternut squash or other squash, finely chopped

½ cup carrots, finely chopped

½ cup cabbage, finely chopped

½ onion, finely chopped

2½ cm (1 inch) piece of wakame

1 shitake mushroom

Miso or shoyu to taste

Chopped scallions or parsley for garnish

Combine all the ingredients except for the seasoning and add three times as much water. Bring to a boil, reduce the flame and let simmer for about 30 minutes. Towards the end of the cooking, season with miso (about half a teaspoon per person) or several drops of shoyu, and simmer for another 3 minutes. Garnish with chopped scallions or parsley.

Clear Shoyu Broth

2 shitake mushrooms

7 cm (3 inch) piece kombu

4 cups water

1 block tofu, cubed

2–3 tbsp shoyu

¼ cup scallions

Nori for garnish

Soak the shitake mushrooms for 20 minutes. Place the kombu and mushrooms in water (include the soaking water) and boil for 5 minutes. Remove the kombu and shitake and save for another recipe. Add the tofu to the pan and boil until it comes to the surface. Do not boil for too long or the tofu will become hard. Add shoyu and simmer for 3 or 4 minutes. Garnish with scallions and pieces of nori.

Barley Soup with Seitan

¼ cup barley

6 cups stock

1 bay leaf

Extra virgin olive oil

2 carrots, thinly sliced

1 onion, finely chopped

1 clove garlic, chopped

1 block seitan

Chopped fresh parsley

Soak the barley overnight and bring two cups of the stock to the boil in a small saucepan. Add the bay leaf and the barley, reduce the heat and simmer for 40 minutes. Heat a small amount of oil in a pan, add the carrots and onions and sauté for about 10 minutes with a clove of chopped garlic. Slice the seitan into small squares and fry in olive oil, until crisp. Add the remaining stock to the carrot and onion and put in the seitan. Reduce the heat, cover and simmer gently for about 20 minutes. Stir in the parsley and serve.

Braised Carrot Soup

4 tsp extra virgin olive oil

1 tbsp balsamic vinegar

1½ tsp sea salt

6–8 carrots, cut into small chunks

½ onion, diced

2 gold potatoes, peeled and diced

4 cups spring water or Dashi Stock (see page 69)

2 sprigs fresh mint, leaves removed and finely shredded

Scant pinch of ground nutmeg

Mint for garnish

Place two teaspoons of the oil, one teaspoon vinegar and half a teaspoon of salt in a large flat-bottomed pan over a medium heat. Arrange the carrots in the oil mixture, avoiding overlap as much as possible. Cover and listen closely for a strong sizzle. When you hear the sizzle, reduce the heat to low and cook until the carrots are tender and the liquid has become a thick syrup – 15 to 20 minutes (depending on the size of the carrot pieces).

Place the remaining two teaspoons of oil and the onion in a large saucepan and cook over a medium heat. When the onion sizzles, add a pinch of salt and sauté for 1 to 2 minutes. Add the potatoes, nutmeg, braised carrots and water. Bring to a boil, cover and reduce heat to low. Cook until the potatoes are tender – about 20 minutes. Season with about one teaspoon of salt and simmer for 5 minutes more. Ladle the soup into a food processor or use a hand blender, and purée until smooth. Serve garnished with mint.

French Onion Soup

1 tbsp extra virgin olive oil

8–10 onions, thinly sliced lengthwise

5 cups spring or filtered water

2 pieces brown rice mochi, cut into ½ cm (¼ inch) cubes

2 tbsp barley miso

2 tbsp minced fresh flat-leaf parsley

Croutons

Pinch of sea salt

Heat the olive oil in a soup pot over a low heat. Add the onions and salt. Cook, stirring occasionally, until lightly browned and reduced in bulk – around 30 minutes. Gently add water and bring to a boil. Reduce the heat, cover and cook for about 15 minutes. Add the mochi cubes. Remove a small amount of broth, add miso and stir until dissolved. Stir back into the soup and simmer for about 5 minutes more, until mochi melts and becomes creamy. Do not boil. Serve garnished with parsley and croutons.

Fresh Corn Chowder

4 ears fresh corn

1 celery stalk, diced

2 onions, diced

5–6 cups water

¼ tsp sea salt

Shoyu to taste

Chopped parsley, watercress or scallions and nori for garnish

Remove the kernels from the corn with a knife. Place the celery, onion and corn in a saucepan. Add water and a pinch of salt. Bring to a boil, lower the flame, cover and simmer until the corn and celery are soft. Add the rest of the salt and shoyu to taste, if desired. Garnish with chopped parsley, watercress or scallions and nori.

Puréed Sweet Vegetable Soup

You will feel relaxed and crave fewer sweets if you add this soup to your diet.

1 onion, cut into large pieces

2 cups squash, cut into large pieces

1 parsnip, cut into large pieces

4–5 cups spring water

2 tsp sea salt

1 cup cabbage, sliced

1 tbsp olive oil

Fresh parsley, torn into pieces

Place the onion, squash and parsnip in a pan and cover with water. Cover with a lid and bring to a boil over a medium flame. Simmer for about 15 minutes and add the sea salt. Simmer a few minutes more and then purée with a hand blender. Add the cabbage and the rest of the water, return to a boil and add the olive oil. Simmer until the cabbage softens slightly and then stir in the parsley.

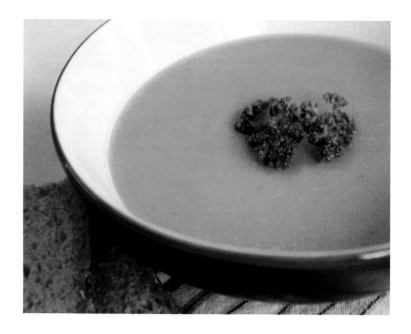

Vegetable Dishes

Braised Cabbage with Umeboshi

½ head white or red cabbage

1 tbsp toasted sesame oil

1½ tbsp umeboshi paste

Cut the cabbage half in two lengthwise. Remove the hard core, and shred the leafy part thinly into ½ cm (¼ inch) slices. Heat the oil over a medium heat in a frying pan, add the cabbage and sauté briefly, stirring with a wooden spoon. Add the umeboshi, which won't mix evenly at first, but as you keep mixing, it will evenly coat the cabbage. Keep cooking like this for 5–10 minutes. After sautéing, if no juice has come out of the cabbage, add a very small drizzle of water, then cover, reduce the heat to low and simmer for 15–20 minutes, or until tender. Serve hot as a side dish with braised tofu or tempeh.

Ginger-Glazed Carrots

2 tsp toasted sesame oil

3 carrots, thinly julienned

1 cup cold water

1 large handful chopped parsley or watercress

1 tsp shoyu

1 heaping tsp kuzu

2 tsp juice squeezed from fresh grated ginger

Pinch of sea salt

Heat the oil in a frying pan, add the carrots and mix with a wooden spoon. Sauté for about 5 minutes. Add the water and salt, cover and simmer over a low heat for 10 minutes, until the carrots are just tender. Add the greens and shoyu, mix together and simmer for 5 minutes. Take the pan off the heat. Dissolve the kuzu in a tablespoon of cold water and slowly add it to the vegetables. Put the pan back on the heat and bring to a simmer while you continue to stir. Cook for another couple of minutes and then add freshly grated ginger juice. Mix and serve as a side dish.

Green Beans Amandine

2 tsp sunflower or safflower oil

½ cup flaked almonds

3 cups green beans, topped and tailed, then thinly sliced

3 tbsp sweet white miso

3 tbsp mirin

Pinch of sea salt

Heat the oil in a medium-sized frying pan over a medium heat. Add the almonds and sauté for 2–3 minutes. Add the green beans and salt, and sauté for 1–2 minutes more. Add enough water to just cover the bottom of the pan. Cover and steam until the beans are tender but still have a crunch. Mix the miso and mirin and pour over the beans. Toss and cook for a minute or two more, adding a little water if needed.

Nishime

Nishime, or water braising of vegetables, calls for large pieces or chunks of root vegetables cooked over low heat until they are tender and sweet. The steam generated by this method of cooking allows the vegetables to cook in their own juices, eliminating the need for anything more than just a little added water. A light seasoning towards the end of cooking brings out their full-bodied flavor and natural sweetness. Vegetables cooked in this manner are quite soft and juicy, giving us a very warming, strengthening energy. A great dish for creating vitality and one to be incorporated into your diet over the long term.

A small piece of kombu in the bottom of the pot brings out the sweetness of the vegetables, naturally tenderizes them by virtue of its glutamic acid and lightly mineralizes the dish, helping to create strong blood.

Nishime-Style Vegetables

Nishime dishes may be very simple, consisting of one root vegetable braised to sweet perfection, or more elaborate, such as hearty stews made up of any number of vegetables. Here is one of my favorites to get you started, with a few suggested variations.

2½ cm (1 inch) piece kombu

2 dried shitake mushrooms, soaked until tender, then thinly sliced

1 carrot, cut into large chunks

1 cup squash, cut into 2½ cm (1 inch) cubes

1 onion, cut into thick wedges

Spring or filtered water

Shoyu sauce

Place the kombu in a heavy pot and either layer the vegetables in the order listed or arrange the vegetables in the pot in individual sections. Add enough water to just cover the bottom of the pot and bring to a boil over a medium heat. Reduce the heat to low, cover and cook until the vegetables are tender – about 25 minutes. Season the vegetables lightly with soy sauce and simmer 10 minutes more, until all the liquid has been absorbed by the vegetables. If the water evaporates too quickly during cooking, add a little more and reduce the heat (because it is cooking too quickly). Transfer to a bowl and serve.

For variety, use Brussels sprouts, leek, parsnip, turnip, green cabbage or whatever vegetables are seasonally available. Opt for organic where possible.

Broccoli with Peanut Sauce

1 large bunch broccoli, separated into florets and stems cut into spears

1 cup smooth peanut butter

¼ cup chopped cilantro

3 tbsp rice syrup

2 tbsp shoyu or tamari

2 tsp cider vinegar

2 small cloves garlic, minced (2 tsp)

sea salt

Bring a large pot of water to the boil, add the broccoli and cook for 2 to 3 minutes, or until bright green and tender. Alternatively, steam the broccoli in a bamboo or wire mesh steamer basket. Drain and rinse the broccoli under cold water to cool. Shake and pat dry. Whisk the peanut butter with one cup of hot water in a bowl. Stir in the remaining ingredients and season with salt. Place the bowl in the center of a serving platter and arrange the broccoli around it.

Sweet French Fries

2 sweet potatoes

Extra virgin olive oil

Sea salt

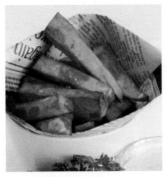

Preheat oven to 230°C/450°F. Slice the potatoes length-wise into one centimeter (half inch) slices, then cut the slices into one centimeter (half inch) spears, just like French fries. Toss them with a generous amount of olive oil to coat well. Spread on a rimmed baking sheet, avoiding overlap, and bake uncovered for about 35 minutes, until browned and crisp. Stir occasionally to ensure even browning. Remove from the oven and toss with a light seasoning of sea salt.

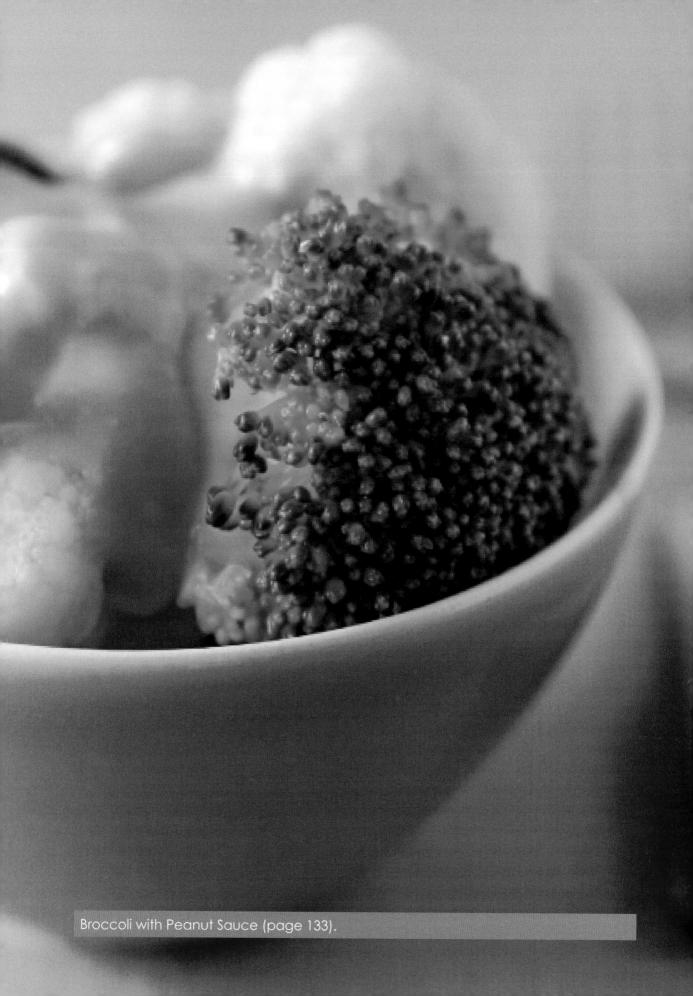

Broccoli with Peanut Sauce (page 133).

Sautéed Vegetables

Sautéed vegetables are quick and delicious, and the energy is perfect for warm weather. But because of the oil, sautéed vegetables are also totally appropriate for colder weather. A great dish for late summer.

1–2 tbsp sesame or olive oil

1 clove garlic, minced

12 mushrooms, sliced

1 cup green beans

Kernels from 1 ear of corn

2 stalks bok choy, cut into 2½ cm (1 inch) pieces

1 tsp shoyu

3 tbsp spring water

Pinch of sea salt

Heat the olive oil over a medium heat in a pan or wok. Add the garlic and salt, stirring constantly for about 10 minutes. Add the mushrooms and stir until they begin to soften. Add the green beans, corn, bok choy and shoyu, stirring to mix everything together. Add the spring water and cover – this small amount of water will steam the vegetables. Cook for 4 minutes. Remove from the heat and serve immediately.

Onion Butter

6 medium onions, sliced into thin half moons

3 tbsp untoasted sesame or olive oil

1 tsp sea salt

Spring water (if needed)

Heat the oil in a cast-iron or enamelled cast-iron pot. Make sure that whatever you use has a heavy lid. Add the onions when the oil is hot and sprinkle with salt to draw out the sweetness and moisture of the onions. Sauté until the onions are translucent (considering the amount of onion, this may take a little while). Add a tiny bit of water if they seem dry or if they are sticking to the bottom of the pot. Cover and reduce the heat to very low, putting a flame deflector under the pot. The heavy lid of the pot will keep all the cooking juices in and the onions should not burn. Simmer for anywhere between 3 and 5 hours, until the onions are completely reduced and really sweet. Serve as a snack, on sourdough bread or rice cakes.

Grain Dishes

Fennel, Mushroom and Almond Risotto

4 cups water

1 sachet (28 g) or 1 tbsp organic bouillon paste

2 tbsp organic extra virgin olive oil

1 small onion, chopped finely

1 clove garlic

1 cup risotto rice

1 tbsp sake

4 fresh shitake mushrooms, chopped finely

½ head fennel, chopped finely

1 pack (35 g)/(¼ cup) of organic tamari roasted almonds, crushed

1 brussels sprout

Bring the water to the boil, add the bouillon and leave on a very low heat for later. Heat the olive oil in a saucepan and add the onion and whole garlic clove with the skin on. Add the rice and cook for 2–3 minutes, stirring continuously. Add the sake and keep stirring until the alcohol has evaporated. Add the shitake mushrooms, fennel and half of the almonds, and cook for 2–3 minutes. Add one ladle of bouillon to the rice and cook at very low heat while stirring continuously. When the bouillon is absorbed, repeat the process until the rice is cooked to your liking. Cover the risotto and leave to rest for a minute. I have simply served this risotto with a drizzle of olive oil and topped with a brussels sprout.

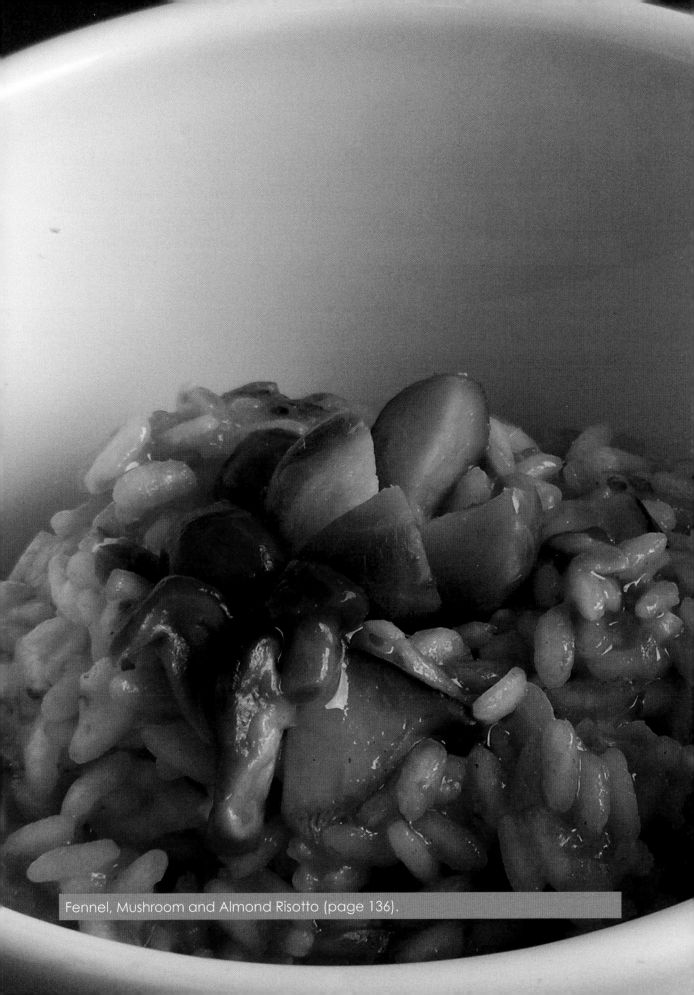

Fennel, Mushroom and Almond Risotto (page 136).

Fruit and Nut Couscous

2 cups water

1 cup wholewheat couscous

⅓ cup dried cranberries

2 tbsp extra virgin olive oil

Juice of ½ lemon

¼ cup slivered almonds, toasted

½ tsp umeboshi plum vinegar

2 tbsp Italian parsley, minced

Sea salt and freshly ground black pepper to taste

Bring the water to a boil over a high heat with a pinch of salt. Add the couscous and boil on a high heat, uncovered, until all the water has been absorbed. Turn off the flame. Scatter the cranberries on top, cover and let sit, undisturbed, for 5 minutes. Fluff with a fork into a large serving bowl. Add in the remaining ingredients and toss well to combine. Add seasoning to taste.

Noodles with Miso-Tahini Sauce

Udon and lo mein noodles go especially well with this popular sauce, and soba noodles are a tasty accompaniment too. Scallions are used as a simple garnish for this version of the recipe, but try topping the noodles and sauce with steamed vegetables.

1 pack uncooked noodles

4 level tbsp sweet white miso

3–4 tbsp tahini

Cold water (for the sauce)

2 tbsp brown rice vinegar

1 tbsp mirin

3 cm (7 inch) piece fresh ginger root, grated and then squeezed for juice

1 clove garlic, finely chopped

Pinch of dried tarragon, basil or thyme

Finely chopped scallion

Boil the noodles in water according to the cooking instructions. Mix the miso and tahini in a small saucepan. Add the water a little at a time, mixing well to make a smooth sauce. Add the remaining ingredients and bring to a gentle simmer. If the sauce is too thick, add a bit more water; if it's too thin, simmer briefly to thicken. To serve, arrange the noodles in individual serving bowls, spoon the sauce over the top and sprinkle with the scallions.

Quinoa with Butternut Squash

2 cups butternut squash, peeled and cubed into small dice

1 tbsp olive oil

1 cup uncooked quinoa

Generous pinch of ground cinnamon

Generous pinch of ground ginger

1⅓ cup bouillon stock

1 tsp sea salt

½ tsp pepper (optional)

In a medium saucepan over a medium heat, add the butternut squash and oil. Sauté until the squash begins to soften slightly (10–15 minutes). Add the quinoa and spices. Lightly toast the quinoa until golden and aromatic – about 1 minute. Add the stock and salt and pepper. Bring to a boil, cover and reduce the heat to low. Cook for 15 minutes, or until the squash is soft and the quinoa is fluffy. Serve immediately.

Millet

Millet is highly nutritious, non-glutinous and, like buckwheat and quinoa, is not an acid-forming food, so is soothing and easy to digest. In fact, it is considered to be one of the least allergenic and most digestible grains available, and it is a warming grain so will help to heat the body in cold or rainy seasons and climates.

Millet is tasty, with a mildly sweet, nutlike flavor, and contains a myriad of beneficial nutrients. It is nearly 15% protein and contains high amounts of fiber, B-complex vitamins (including niacin, thiamine and riboflavin), methionine (an essential amino acid), lecithin and some vitamin E. It is particularly high in the minerals iron, magnesium, phosphorous and potassium. Millet is delicious as a cooked cereal and as an ingredient in casseroles, breads, soups, stews, soufflés, pilaf and stuffing. It can be served as a side dish or under sautéed vegetables or with beans, and can be popped like corn for use as a snack or breakfast cereal. The grain mixes well with any seasoning or herbs that are commonly used in rice dishes, and for interesting taste and texture variations it may be combined with quinoa or brown rice.

Millet may also be sprouted for use in salads and sandwiches. The seeds are also rich in phytochemicals, including phytic acid, which is believed to lower cholesterol, and phytates, which are associated with reduced cancer risk.

Steamed Millet

This recipe is as basic as steamed rice and, like rice, its variations are endless. Using it to exemplify "Cook once – eat twice," notice how one pot of millet can form the basis of several meals in a row.

1 cup millet

2¼ cups water or stock

1 tsp extra virgin olive oil

¼ tsp sea salt

Rinse the millet and drain in a strainer. Place in a saucepan, add the water, oil and salt, and bring to a boil. Reduce the heat, cover and simmer for about 20 minutes, or until all the water has been absorbed. Turn off the heat and let stand, covered, for 5 minutes. Fluff the millet with a fork and serve.

✿ Spoon hot millet into a shallow pan, smooth the top and allow to cool. Slice into wedges and bake or fry as polenta.

✿ As a side dish, serve freshly cooked millet with a condiment, chutney or sauce.

✿ Stir fry millet with tempeh or tofu.

✿ Shape millet into a croquette with chopped herbs and, if necessary, some flour to bind it and pan fry or bake (alternatively bind with tofu). Or form into a casserole, top with a jar of organic tomato sauce and bake.

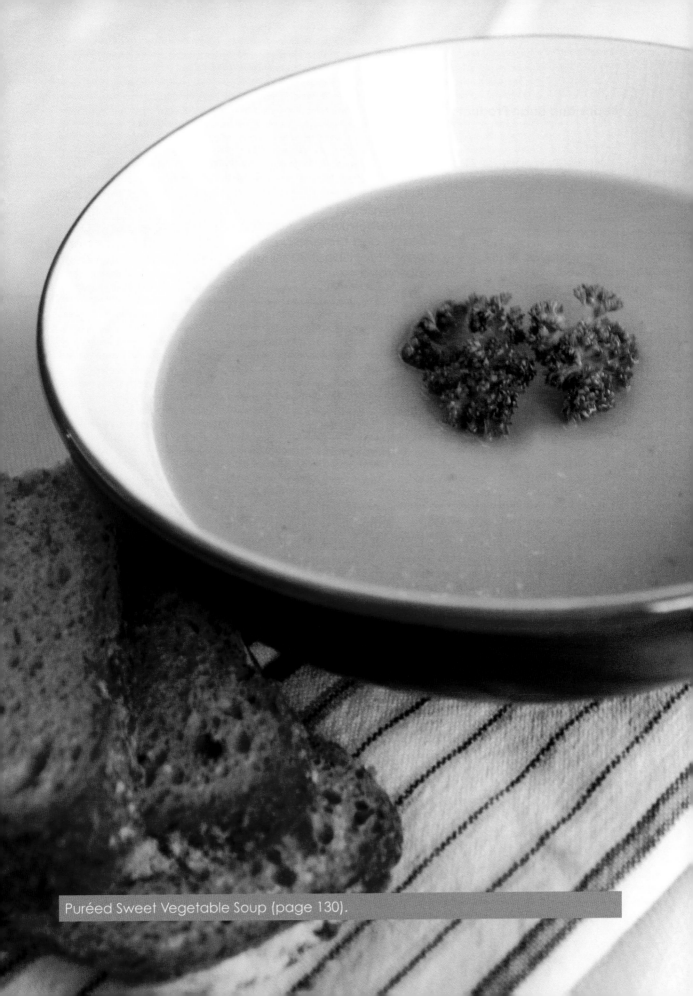

Puréed Sweet Vegetable Soup (page 130).

Beans and Bean Products

Lentil Pilaf

2 tbsp olive oil

1 bunch scallions, chopped

2 garlic cloves, finely chopped

1 cup lentils, rinsed

½ cup brown rice, rinsed

½ cup wild rice, rinsed

2 tbsp flaked almonds

½ tsp dried thyme

3 cups Dashi Stock (see page 69)

In a large saucepan, sauté the onions, garlic, lentils and both types of rice in the olive oil until the onion is tender – about 5 minutes. Add the almonds, thyme and Dashi Stock, and bring to a boil. Reduce the heat, cover and simmer for about 30 minutes, or until the liquid has been absorbed.

Chickpea Stew

A thick and creamy stew that is a meal on its own. Make enough for dinner and save the leftovers for tomorrow's lunch, served with some fresh greens.

1 onion, finely diced

1 clove fresh garlic, finely minced

5 cups Dashi Stock (see page 69)

Fresh corn, if available, or canned or frozen corn

Jar or can of cooked chickpeas (natural food store)

Green cabbage, finely shredded

2 tsp white miso

Extra virgin olive oil

Parsley for garnish

Combine the onion, garlic and a small amount of stock in a soup pot over a medium heat. Bring to a boil, reduce the heat and simmer for 5 minutes. Add the remaining stock and return to a boil. Stir in the corn, chickpeas and cabbage, cover and cook over a low heat for about 50 minutes, stirring occasionally. Remove a small amount of broth with a cup and add miso and stir until it is dissolved. Stir the mixture back into the pot and simmer for 5 minutes – do not boil miso or you will destroy the precious enzymes. Serve, drizzled with olive oil and garnished with some fresh parsley.

Pasta with Sweet and Sour Tempeh and Pumpkin

250 g (9 oz) penne pasta

1 pack fresh tempeh, cut into cubes

Sunflower oil for deep frying

2 tbsp shoyu

2 tbsp mirin

1 tbsp brown rice vinegar

½ tbsp olive oil

1 onion, sliced

1 garlic clove, chopped finely

½ tsp ginger powder or 2½ cm (1 inch) piece of fresh ginger, grated or finely chopped

1 sweet pumpkin (red/ green Hokkaido) or butternut squash, cubed

1 tsp oregano

Sea salt

Cook the pasta in boiling water with a pinch of sea salt for 10–12 minutes, then rinse under cold water to stop it cooking any further and set aside. Deep fry the tempeh until golden in color and drain on paper towels. Put the shoyu, mirin and brown rice vinegar in a saucepan, add the tempeh and simmer. Reduce until all the liquid has been absorbed then set the tempeh aside. Gently fry the onion in olive oil for 3 minutes, add a pinch of salt and the garlic and ginger, and continue cooking for 2 minutes. Add the pumpkin and oregano and a little water, cover and simmer until the pumpkin is soft (approximately 15 minutes). Blend the onion, garlic and pumpkin with a stick blender, adding enough water to make a thick sauce. Add the tempeh and pasta to the pumpkin and stir. Serve with steamed greens, such as kale, spring greens or broccoli.

Adzuki Bean Pâté

1 cup adzuki beans

2 cups water

1 piece kombu

1 onion, chopped fine

1 cup mushrooms, chopped

1–2 cloves garlic, chopped fine

Dill

Tamari

Soak the adzuki beans overnight. (Alternatively, simply use the leftover beans from the Sweet and Sour Adzuki Bean recipe, page 208.) Drain and rinse the beans well, then place them in a pot with two cups of water and the kombu (broken up into pieces). Bring to a boil, turn down the heat to low and cook until done. Sauté the onions and add the mushrooms. Add garlic to taste. Add dill and tamari to taste. Place the beans in a blender and purée until smooth, adding water if necessary. Add the onions and mushrooms. A great dip for celery, cucumbers, radishes, and cauliflower, or spread on wholegrain toast or crackers.

Sauces, Salads and Side Dishes

Wakame and Cucumber Salad

4 heaping tbsp wakame flakes

2 baby cucumbers or 1 regular cucumber, cut into wafer-thin slices

½ tsp sea salt

Fresh ginger (about 5 cm/2 inch piece), peeled and cut into thin shreds

4–6 tbsp Miso and Sweet Vinegar Dressing (see below)

Soak the wakame in a bowl of cold water for 15 minutes. Soak the cucumbers in a bowl of cold water with the sea salt for 10 minutes. Drain both well. Place the wakame and cucumbers in a bowl, add the ginger and drizzle with Miso and Sweet Vinegar Dressing. Toss well and serve.

Miso and Sweet Vinegar Dressing

This is delicious as a salad dressing or drizzled over vegetables.

2 tbsp sake

½ pack (125 g) white miso paste

½ cup brown rice vinegar

3 tbsp rice malt syrup

Put the sake in a small saucepan and bring to the boil over a medium heat to burn off the alcohol, then reduce the heat to low. Add the other ingredients and stir well with a wooden spoon, simmering for a few minutes. Remove from the heat and allow to cool to room temperature. Store in a glass jar and refrigerate – it can be kept for up to 4 weeks. It has a strong taste, so drizzle sparingly as only a little is required to liven up your dishes.

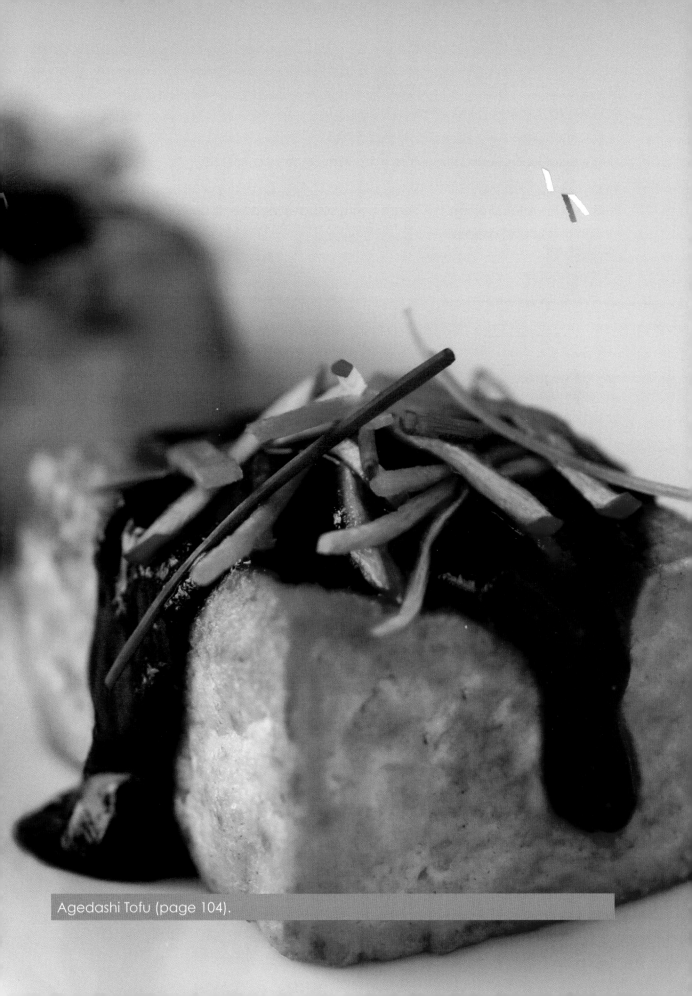

Agedashi Tofu (page 104).

Chunky Artichoke and Chickpea Salad

For a tasty lunch, serve this dish as a dip with crackers or spread.

1 jar artichoke hearts packed in water, drained

1 can chickpeas, drained and rinsed

¼ cup chopped onion

¼ cup chopped baby pickles

¼ cup chopped fresh celery

¼ cup vegan mayonnaise

2 tsp olive oil

1 tsp capers

1 clove garlic, minced (1 tsp)

1 tsp Dijon mustard

Pulse all the ingredients in a food processor until chunky. Season with salt and pepper, if desired. Chill for at least 30 minutes, or overnight. Serve with fresh green salad and some crackers.

Warm Salad with Sautéed Mushrooms

Mixture of salad leaves

1 tbsp olive oil

1–2 shallots, sliced

6 fresh shitake mushrooms, quartered and torn

1 tbsp mirin

1 tbsp shoyu

Fresh tarragon leaves, chopped

Toasted pumpkin seeds

Gomashio (see page 116)

Prepare a bowl of exotic lettuce leaves, arugula, watercress, or spinach. Heat a little oil in a frying pan and fry the shallots till soft. Add a handful of fresh shitake mushrooms, as necessary, and fry for a few minutes. Add one tablespoon of mirin and one tablespoon of shoyu, and a few chopped fresh tarragon leaves. Fry for another 10 seconds or so, then pile onto the salad leaves. Serve immediately, topped with toasted pumpkin seeds and a sprinkling of gomashio.

Soba and Slaw Salad with Peanut Dressing

1 pack uncooked soba noodles

2 cups shredded red cabbage

1 cup shredded green cabbage

1 cup grated carrots

Peanut Dressing

3 tbsp soy sauce

2 tbsp brown rice vinegar

1 tbsp avocado or olive oil

3 cloves fresh garlic, finely minced

3 tbsp creamy peanut butter

3 tbsp dry toasted pumpkin seeds

3 fresh scallions, thinly sliced on the diagonal

2 tbsp unsweetened soy or almond milk

Bring a pot of water to a boil and cook the soba al dente – about 10 minutes. Drain and rinse well with filtered water then transfer to a mixing bowl. Mix in the cabbage and shredded carrots and set aside.

Make the peanut dressing by combining all dressing ingredients in a saucepan over a medium-low heat, slowly whisking in soy milk to make the dressing richer. Cook, stirring constantly, until the sauce is smooth and well blended – about 3 minutes. Gently mix the sauce into the noodles and vegetables. Transfer to a serving platter and sprinkle with pumpkin seeds and scallions.

Shitake Gravy

Pour this delicious gravy over all your favorite grain dishes.

500 ml (2 cups) water for soaking

2 shitake mushrooms, soaked and sliced (reserve soaking water)

2 tbsp extra virgin olive oil

2 cloves garlic, chopped

1 small onion, diced

3 tbsp wholewheat flour

1 tbsp shoyu

1 tbsp mirin

½ tsp dried thyme

Heat the oil in a small pan and sauté the mushrooms, garlic and onion over a medium-low heat for about 5 minutes, until the onion is translucent. Lower the heat, sprinkle the flour over the vegetables, and stir constantly for 2–3 minutes. Slowly add the soaking water while stirring with a wooden spoon, to stop the flour from going lumpy. Keep stirring until the gravy begins to simmer and thicken. Add the shoyu, mirin and thyme, and simmer gently for 15 minutes, stirring now and again. Keep warm until you are ready to serve.

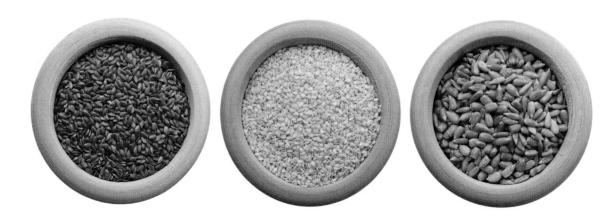

Creamy Sesame Dressing

4 rounded tbsp toasted sesame tahini

2 tbsp onion, chopped

2 umeboshi plums, pitted and chopped

2 tbsp brown rice syrup or barley malt

1 cup spring or filtered water

Dash of soy sauce

Combine all the ingredients in a blender and purée until smooth, slowly adding water to achieve a creamy consistency.

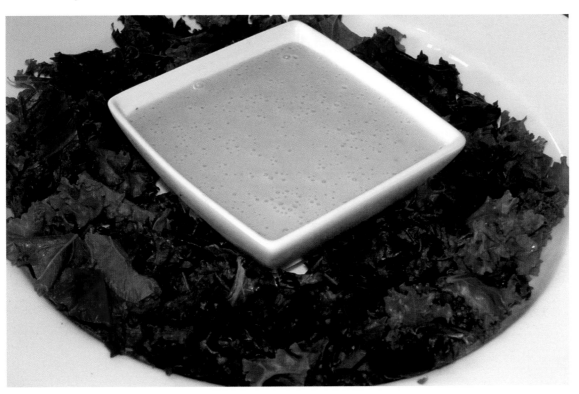

Baked Wakame with Onion and Squash

2 cups onion, sliced into thin half moons

1 cup wakame, soaked and sliced into 5 cm (2 inch) pieces (reserve soaking water)

2 tbsp sesame tahini

1 tsp shoyu

½ small butternut squash, thinly sliced (unpeeled if organic)

Preheat oven to 180°C/350°F. Place the onion in a saucepan with a small amount of wakame soaking water. Bring to a boil, cover, reduce the flame and simmer for 5 minutes. Remove and place in a small casserole dish. Mix the wakame with the onion. Dilute the tahini with about half a cup of wakame soaking water and the shoyu, and mix with the wakame and onion. Smooth the mixture evenly in a casserole dish and layer the sliced squash over the top till covered. Cover and bake in the oven for 30 minutes. Remove the cover and bake for another 10–15 minutes, to remove excess liquid and slightly brown the top.

Desserts

Vanilla Dessert

2 cups plain, vanilla or almond rice milk

½ cup rice malt syrup

2 level tbsp agar-agar flakes

1½ tbsp kuzu, crushed

1 tsp vanilla extract

Berries in season

Pinch of sea salt

Combine one and a half cups of the rice milk with the malt syrup and salt in a small saucepan. Sprinkle in the agar-agar flakes and bring to a simmer over a medium heat. Simmer for 1 minute while stirring. Thoroughly dissolve the kuzu in the remaining rice milk and add to the mix while stirring briskly. Return to a simmer and cook for 1 to 2 minutes. Remove from the heat. Mix in the vanilla extract and leave to set in a glass dish in the refrigerator. (As a variation, for a lemon dessert you can add one and a half tablespoons of lemon juice and one and a half teaspoons of lightly grated lemon zest along with the vanilla.) Purée in a blender to a smooth cream and divide among four small dessert cups. Top with fruit berries.

Baked Apples with Toasted Walnuts

4 large apples, such as Gala or Granny Smith, halved crosswise and cored

2 tsp lemon juice, divided

2 tbsp maple sugar

¼ tsp ground cinnamon

1 cup maple syrup

⅛ tsp salt

½ cup chopped toasted walnuts

Preheat oven to 200°C/400°F. Brush the cut sides of the apples with one teaspoon of lemon juice. Arrange the apples, cut sides up, in a baking dish. Combine the maple sugar and cinnamon in a small bowl and sprinkle the cut sides of the apples with the sugar mixture. Pour the maple syrup into the bottom of the baking dish. Cover with foil and bake for 10 minutes. Uncover and bake for 15 minutes more, or until the apples are tender. Transfer the apples to a serving platter. Pour the syrup and pan juices into a small saucepan and stir in the remaining one teaspoon of lemon juice and salt. Bring to a boil and cook for 2 minutes, or until the sauce is thickened, whisking constantly. Stir in the walnuts. Spoon the sauce over the apples and serve warm.

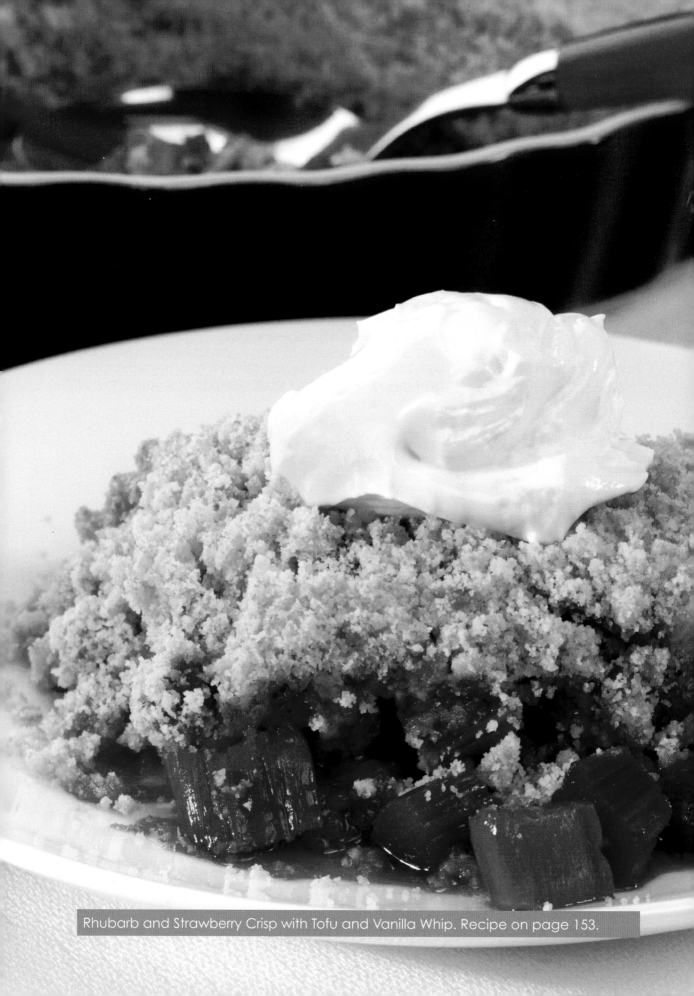

Rhubarb and Strawberry Crisp with Tofu and Vanilla Whip. Recipe on page 153.

Rhubarb and Strawberry Crisp

Serve on its own or with Tofu and Vanilla Whip (see below) or Almond Cream (see page 120).

Rhubarb, chopped (about 6 cups)

1 cup organic apple or white grape juice

2 tbsp rice malt syrup

1 tsp cinnamon

3 tbsp arrowroot powder

1 basket (250 g) strawberries, hulled and quartered (about 2 cups)

2 cups rolled oats

½ cup hazelnut or almond flour

½ tsp cinnamon

⅔ cup maple sugar

½ cup safflower or sunflower oil

Pinch of sea salt

Preheat oven to 200°C/400°F. Combine the rhubarb, three-quarters of a cup of apple juice, rice malt syrup and cinnamon in a saucepan. Bring to a boil, reduce the heat and simmer for 5 minutes. Dissolve the arrowroot in the remaining quarter cup of juice. Add to the rhubarb and cook for 3 minutes. Remove pan from the heat, cool slightly and add the strawberries. Pour the fruit into a 20×20 cm (8×8–inch) glass baking dish and set aside. Combine oats, nut flour, cinnamon, maple sugar and a pinch of salt in a mixing bowl. Add oil and mix thoroughly. Sprinkle the crisp topping over the fruit and bake for 20 minutes, or until golden brown. Serve warm or at room temperature.

Tofu and Vanilla Whip

This simple, creamy dessert sauce keeps for several days and can be used in place of whipped cream with fruit, cakes or tarts.

1 pack silken tofu

⅓ cup maple syrup

1 tbsp olive, sunflower or safflower oil

1 tbsp soy milk

1½ tsp vanilla extract

1 tsp lemon juice

Pinch of sea salt

Whip all the ingredients together in a food processor or blender until very smooth. Refrigerate for at least two hours before serving.

Chapter 9

FIGHTING FIT FOR AUTUMN

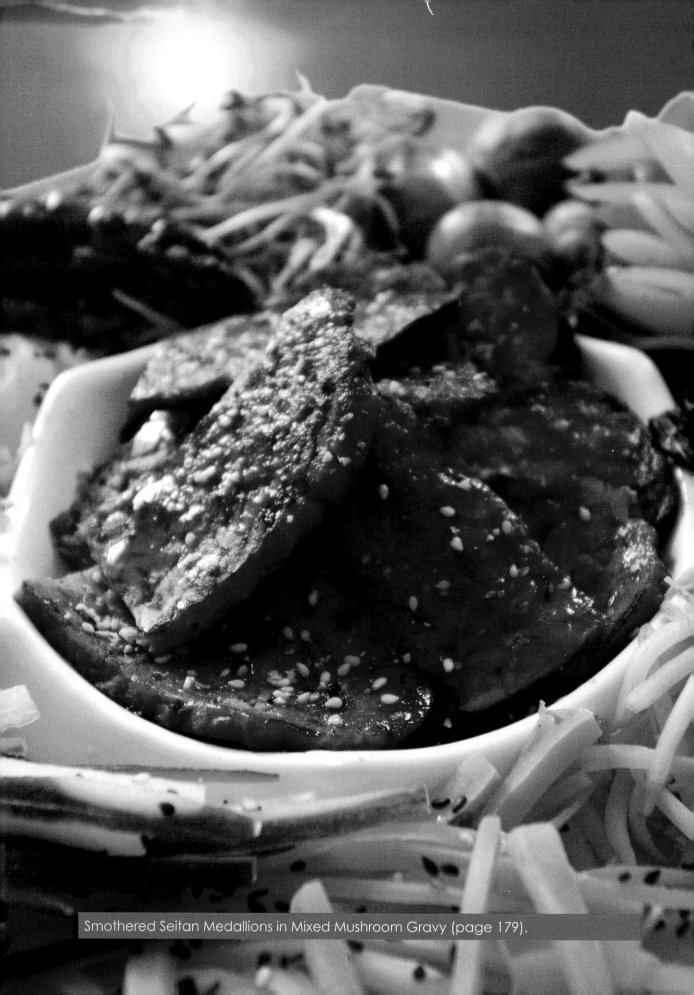

Smothered Seitan Medallions in Mixed Mushroom Gravy (page 179).

As I mentioned earlier, autumn is my earliest recollection of feeling the connection with nature; I was also born in the autumn. It is the season during which both my sister and my dad passed away, and it is the season when energy settles into the earth. The leaves fall from the trees and everything stops growing. The life-giving light of the spring and the summer begins to wane, and the vigorous energy of those seasons comes to an end. There is a beautiful sadness to autumn.

As a child, one of my fondest memories of this season was watching the farmers bringing in their harvest; the hard work that they had painstakingly struggled with during the many months since the spring had now come to fruition. Seeing the large bales of hay being stacked in the fields in neat rows makes a pretty picture. When we visited the country we used to go to the harvest festivals where we would all take huge baskets of fruits, vegetables and food to give to the sick or the poor.

Chestnuts would fall from the trees and nourish us in many ways. Roasting them over an open fire was a delicious way to enjoy them. Or we would amuse ourselves for hours on end playing games with them, by piercing a hole in the chestnut and threading through a piece of string, and challenging an opponent to endless games that we'd make up. That was an autumn event in my neighborhood.

General Considerations

As temperatures fall and the evenings draw in, our motivation to exercise is less apparent. It is important though to stretch out the muscles of the body and get plenty of aerobic exercise. Breath is your life!

The corresponding organs for the METAL element are the lungs and large intestine. The lungs expel carbon dioxide, and the large intestine eliminates solid residue. If these wastes are not eliminated frequently, the skin can be affected. The skin is sometimes referred to as the "third lung" – it is part of the METAL element and can reflect sluggish bowels. The bowels are one of the most important routes of elimination for self-cleansing and work together with the kidneys, bladder, lungs and skin to help eliminate waste efficiently from the body.

In nature, autumn reflects dryness: when the leaves lose their moisture, they shrivel up and "let go" of the branches they have hung on to since springtime. It is therefore the time to reflect on the past year and to prepare to withdraw as the winter months close in. It is very important to protect the back of the neck from the wind, which is gradually getting colder, otherwise you will be more susceptible to minor illnesses after the summer months. If there is an imbalance in the lungs, you can experience breathing difficulties; this indicates that there are unresolved issues connected to the emotion of grief, which corresponds to the METAL element.

Something Like Autumn

Autumn is the time of the lungs. Coughs, colds and sore throats are all connected to problems with METAL energy. There are some special drinks listed below for healing the lungs but one of the principal foods for healthy lungs are leafy green vegetables. Adding a little ginger, garlic and radish to your food can stimulate the lungs. A hot compress such as a ginger compress or a mustard plaster can stimulate the energy in stagnant lungs.

Doing exercises that open up the chest and shoulder areas can get the lung energy moving again, as well as breathing exercises. It seems so silly to say it, but if you want to get healthy lungs there is one thing you must do – breathe! Doing aerobic exercises, such as fast walking, bicycling and swimming, is great.

Special Drinks and Home Remedies

Lotus Root Tea

Using fresh lotus root or lotus root powder to relieve lung congestion and coughs is a winner. This tea is great to soothe a sore throat.

1 tsp lotus root per serving	Add the lotus root to the water and stir to dissolve. Add a pinch of sea salt or a few drops of shoyu. You may also add a couple of drops of grated ginger juice, if desired. Heat on a low flame but do not boil. Turn off the heat when the liquid begins to simmer. Drink while hot.
1 cup water	
Sea salt or shoyu	
Ginger juice (optional)	

Fresh Carrot, Celery and Ginger Juice

Carrot removes the energy downwards from the throat, celery moves energy upwards and the ginger moves the energy out. Use equal parts of carrots and celery and a tiny piece of ginger, and juice in a juicer.

For congestion in the lungs ...

... try steamed greens and ginger – the steamed greens move energy up and the ginger moves energy out. Steam the greens until vibrant green and then squeeze some freshly grated ginger juice on top. Sprinkle with gomashio (see page 116). Also, try parsley tea – the parsley moves energy up and out.

Sesame Seed Tea

1 tbsp slightly crushed sesame seeds

1 tbsp ground linseed

1 cup water

Natural sweetener or salt to taste

Add the sesame seeds and linseed to one cup of boiling water and simmer for 15 minutes. If you prefer a sweet taste, add a teaspoon of a natural sweetener, such as rice syrup or barley malt. For a salty taste, add a drop of shoyu. Take daily for 2 to 3 weeks. Drink the seeds as well as the liquid. To relieve constipation try this tea using black or brown sesame seeds.

To relieve bloating ...

... try root vegetable soups and stews – the roots and cooking style move energy down. Use carrots, parsnips, burdock or daikon / mooli and add some chopped fennel to the cut pieces of root vegetables you are using. Place in a pan and cover with water, bring to a boil and simmer for 30 minutes. Add a few drops of tamari towards the end of cooking.

Bancha Tea with Shoyu and Scallions

For a cold-relief drink, add hot water to a bancha tea bag, a splash of shoyu and a teaspoon of diced scallions.

To relieve a cold ...

... try miso soup with leafy greens. Follow the instructions for the Autumn Miso Soup recipe in this chapter (see page 160) and add some leafy greens at the end of cooking. Simmer for a few minutes until the greens wilt.

Hot Ginger and Lemon Tea

Another great tea for relieving a cold. Grate some fresh ginger, squeeze the juice into a mug of hot water and add a squeeze of lemon juice.

Recipes for Autumn

(Each recipe yields 4 servings)

Soups

> *Miso*
>
> *Miso is a fermented soybean paste used to flavor various dishes, but most widely as a stock to season soups. Miso's natural fermentation process creates a combination of enzymes that strengthen and nourish the intestinal tract. As a result, the blood that nourishes the balance of the body is much stronger. The quality of our blood creates the people we are and the health we possess. Miso has been used for centuries in the Orient as a remedy for cancer, weak digestion, low libido, several types of intestinal infections, high cholesterol, and so much more, and is one of the world's most medicinal foods.*

Autumn Miso Soup

This basic miso soup should be a daily staple of your diet. It encompasses the use of sea vegetables to mineralize the blood, and a variety of fresh vegetables. The balance of these ingredients creates a strengthening energy, vital to life.

12 cm (5 inch) piece of kombu

2 dried shitake or maitake mushrooms

Spring or filtered water

1 piece of wakame

1 onion, diced

1 carrot, diced

1 celery stick, diced

1 tsp miso per cup of soup

Scallions, finely diced, for garnish

Soak the kombu and dried mushrooms in 1½ liters (2½ pints) of spring or filtered water for 30 minutes. Remove the mushrooms (discard the stem as it can be bitter tasting), dice them and place back in the pot. Bring the stock to a boil then lower the heat and simmer for 10 minutes. (This stock is called *dashi* in Japan and is the base for many noodle dishes, stews and sauces, as well as soups). Soak the wakame for 10 minutes and then cut into small pieces with kitchen scissors. Add the wakame and the soaking water to the pot and simmer for 10 minutes.

Add the rest of the vegetables to the pot and bring back to a boil then simmer for 20 minutes. Whisk the miso with a little of the broth and then add to the soup and simmer for 3 minutes. Do not allow the miso to boil or it will destroy the enzymes. Serve hot, with finely chopped scallions to garnish. You can add cubed tofu or soba noodles to make the soup more of a meal.

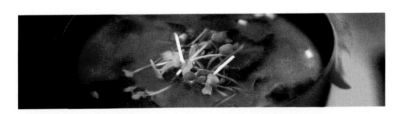

Barley Soup (Stew)

1 small onion or leek, sliced

½ cup corn kernels

½ cup barley

5–6 cups water

Shoyu to taste

Chopped scallions or nori pieces

Layer the ingredients with the onions on the bottom, the corn in the middle and the barley on top. Cook gently until the barley is done – about 45 minutes. Towards the end of cooking, add shoyu to taste. Garnish with chopped scallions or nori pieces.

Italian Minestrone

A delicious, warming and nourishing soup for the cooler days of autumn. Use Dashi Stock to add richness to the flavor as well as gaining the benefits of incredible minerals from the kombu.

1 tbsp extra virgin olive oil

2–3 cloves fresh garlic, finely minced

1 large onion, finely diced

2–3 celery stalks, finely diced

2–3 ripe tomatoes, coarsely chopped (or can of organic chopped tomatoes)

1 large carrot, diced

Generous pinch of dried basil

¼ cup each chickpeas, kidney beans, white beans (use organic, either canned or from a jar)

4 cups Dashi Stock (see page 69)

1 bay leaf

1 cup tiny pasta (short-cut macaroni or look for a quinoa pasta or similar in size), cooked al dente and then rinsed

Several leaves of parsley, finely diced

Grated Parmesan cheese (dairy free)

Sea salt

Heat the oil in a soup pot over a medium-low heat. Add the garlic and onion and a pinch of sea salt, and cook for about 3 minutes. Add celery, tomatoes, carrot, basil and a generous pinch of sea salt. (I prefer to use canned, chopped organic tomatoes as they give the soup a richer tomato taste.) Cook, stirring until coated with oil.

Add all the beans, four cups of Dashi Stock and a bay leaf. Bring to a boil, cover and simmer over a low heat for about 30 minutes, adding more Dashi Stock if required for a thinner consistency. Season with another pinch of sea salt and then simmer for 10 more minutes. Remove the bay leaf, stir in the cooked pasta and simmer a few minutes more. Serve hot, garnished with fresh parsley and grated Parmesan cheese if you so desire.

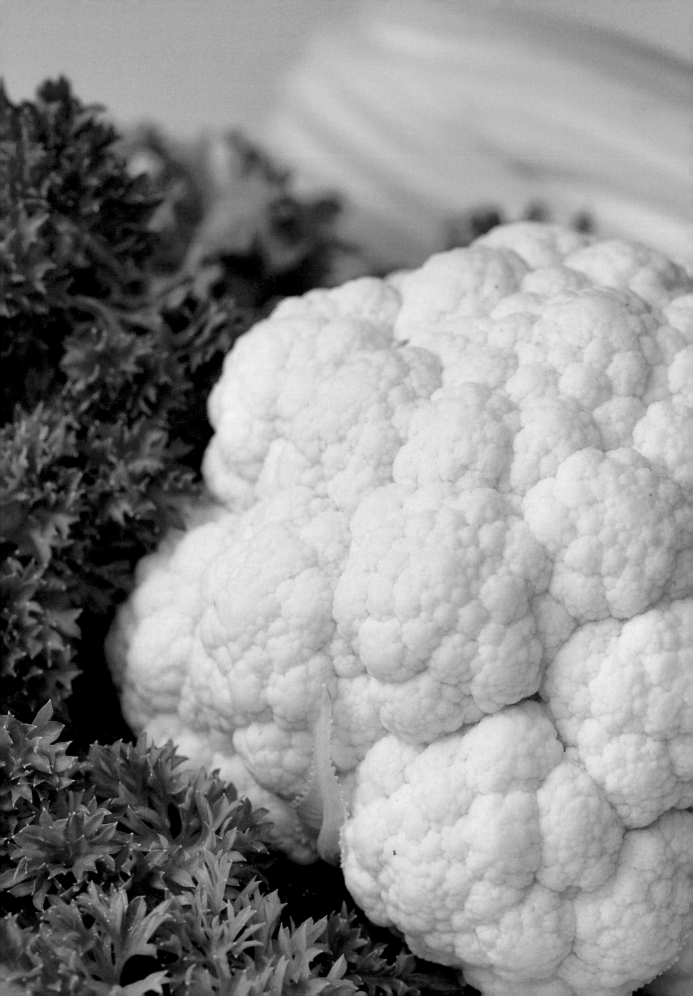

Cauliflower Soup

1 large cauliflower, green part removed and discarded

1 large onion, chopped

2 potatoes, peeled and diced

2 cloves garlic, diced

3 cups Dashi Stock (see page 69)

1 cup soy milk

2 cups water

½ cup herbs, chopped (tarragon works well)

1 tbsp tamari or shoyu

Pinch sea salt

Scallions, finely sliced

Toasted black sesame seeds for garnish

Cut the cauliflower in half and pull off the florets. Place the cauliflower, onion, potatoes and garlic in a pot and add three cups of Dashi Stock. Bring to a boil and then simmer for 20 minutes. Add one cup of soy milk and two cups of water, along with some chopped herbs of your choice and the tamari. Cook for 10 minutes and then season with a pinch of sea salt and simmer 5 minutes more. Blend with a hand blender and serve in warmed bowls. Add some scallions and black sesame seeds for garnish. Season with salt and pepper if desired.

Leek, Potato and Onion Soup

2 tbsp olive oil

4 large leeks, washed

1 large onion

2 large potatoes

6 cups Dashi Stock (see page 69)

Chopped chives

Chop and slice all the vegetables. Heat the oil in a large pan and add the vegetables. Sweat over a low heat with the lid on for about 20 minutes. Add the stock and bring to the boil, lower the heat and simmer for 20 minutes. Blend with a hand blender and serve with chopped chives.

Lentil Soup

1 bunch of kale or other greens

1 large carrot

1 large onion

1 clove of garlic

3 tbsp olive oil

Sea salt

1 cup green lentils

4 cups Dashi Stock (see page 69)

Purée the greens, carrot, onion and garlic in a food processor. Heat the oil in a heavy-based pan and add the vegetables. Sauté and sweat for 5 minutes and then add some sea salt. Place the green lentils into the pot and add the Dashi Stock. Bring to a boil and simmer for 45 minutes. Either blend to a creamy soup or serve chunky as a hearty soup.

Chickpea, Chard and Couscous Soup

The greens with the couscous are a really nice combination.

Olive oil

1 onion, finely diced

2 garlic cloves, minced

1 tsp dried thyme

1 can chickpeas, rinsed and drained

½ cup couscous

1 large bunch chard or kale, leaves cut off the stems and cut or torn into bite-size pieces

6 cups light vegetable stock or bouillon

Heat a large pot over medium heat and add just enough olive oil to coat the bottom of the pot. Add the onions and cook until they begin to soften – about 5 minutes. Add the garlic and thyme and stir for 2 minutes. Add the chickpeas and the couscous and cook for 2–3 minutes, stirring often to keep the couscous from sticking to the bottom of the pan. Add the chard, in batches if need be, and stir well to combine. Pour in the vegetable stock and bring to a boil. Reduce the heat and allow the soup to simmer for about 30 minutes – enough time for the couscous to cook, the greens to soften and the flavors to blend.

Creamy Mushroom Soup

Handful mixed dried mushrooms, such as oyster, maitake, porcini and chanterelles

1½ cups vegetable broth or bouillon

¼ cup rice mirin

1 tbsp olive oil, divided

½ tsp sea salt

Fresh mushrooms, such as shitake and white button, chopped (2 cups)

½ cup finely chopped scallions

¼ tsp ground black pepper (optional)

1 clove garlic, minced (1 tsp)

1 tbsp all-purpose flour

½ cup oat milk or other non-dairy milk

Place dried mushrooms in a medium bowl. Cover with 2 cups of hot water and let stand for 30 minutes. Drain the mushrooms, reserving the soaking liquid. Bring the soaking liquid, broth and rice mirin to a simmer in a saucepan over a medium heat. Cover and keep warm.

Heat one teaspoon of oil in a saucepan over a medium heat. Add the rehydrated mushrooms and one-quarter of a teaspoon of salt. Sauté for 2 minutes, or until the mushrooms are tender. Transfer the mushrooms to a plate and set aside.

Heat the remaining one teaspoon of oil in the same saucepan over a medium heat. Add the fresh mushrooms, scallions, pepper and remaining quarter of a teaspoon of salt. Cook for 2 minutes, stirring frequently. Add the garlic and cook for 30 seconds, or until fragrant. Increase the heat to medium-high and simmer for 3 minutes, or until the liquid is reduced by half. Whisk the flour into the broth mixture. Stir the broth mixture into the mushroom mixture, and bring to a boil. Reduce the heat to medium-low and simmer for 30 minutes. Transfer the soup to a blender or food processor and purée until smooth. Return the soup to the pot and stir in the milk and the set-aside rehydrated mushrooms – reserve a few for garnish, if desired. Serve in bowls garnished with a swirl of tamari and flaked almonds.

Vegetable Dishes

Greens with Japanese Vinaigrette

Lightly cooked greens are full of vibrant color and concentrated goodness. The simple dressing in this recipe complements the slightly bitter flavor of the greens. Carrots and sesame seeds add a great contrast of color and texture.

1 large bunch leafy greens, e.g. kale or spring greens

1 medium carrot, julienned

1 tbsp toasted sesame oil

1 tbsp brown rice vinegar

1 tbsp shoyu

1 tbsp sesame seeds, toasted

1 tbsp pumpkin seeds, toasted

Wash the greens and remove any tough stems or damaged bits from the leaves. Steam until the greens are tender then remove from the pot. Steam the carrots for 4–5 minutes. Drain and set aside. In a small bowl, whisk together the oil, vinegar and shoyu with a fork. Toss the greens and carrots in a mixing bowl with the dressing. Serve sprinkled with the sesame and pumpkin seeds.

Glazed Carrots

2 large carrots, cut into small irregular pieces

7 cm (3 inch) piece wakame, soaked until tender and thinly sliced

½ tsp light sesame oil

2 tbsp barley malt

2 tbsp rice syrup

Slivered almonds, lightly pan toasted, for garnish

Sea salt

Bring a large pot of water to a boil with a pinch of sea salt. Add the carrots and cook until just tender – about 5 minutes. Remove with a strainer and cook the wakame pieces in the same water for 5 to 7 minutes. Drain and toss with the carrots. Set aside while preparing the glaze.

To prepare the glaze, bring the oil, barley malt and rice syrup with a generous pinch of salt to a boil in a small saucepan over a medium heat, cooking until foamy. Stir the glaze into the carrots and kombu until well coated. Transfer to a serving bowl and garnish generously with slivered almonds.

Autumn Roasted Vegetables

1 leek, washed and sliced into 2½ cm (1 inch) pieces

2 parsnips, chunked

1 cup cubed Hokkaido or butternut squash

Dried thyme and sage

Olive oil

Sea salt

Spring water

Preheat oven to 180°C/350°F. Mix all the above ingredients together and drizzle with olive oil and sea salt. Add a small amount of water to the baking tray, cover with foil and bake for 45 to 60 minutes.

Sautéed Vegetables

Leafy greens and thickly sliced root vegetables, as well as sprouts or corn kernels may all be sautéed by themselves or in various combinations.

Sesame oil

Assortment of organic seasonal vegetables, finely sliced

Sea salt or shoyu to taste

Heat a pan and add a small volume of sesame oil. When the oil is hot, sauté the vegetables quickly for a few minutes. Gently stir the vegetables with chopsticks or a wooden spoon. There is no need for vigorous stirring or constant mixing. Sprinkle with a pinch of sea salt or shoyu. Simmer for a few more minutes, adding a little water if necessary. The vegetables should be crispy and colorful, and cooked, but not overcooked. The cooking time may vary depending on the type, size and thickness of the ingredients. Serve with one of the sauces on pages 181–183 and sprinkle with chia seeds.

Baked Pumpkin with Onion Gravy

Olive oil

7–8 onions, finely cut into half moons

3–4 bay leaves

1 tbsp white miso

2–3 tbsp mirin

1 tbsp kuzu

½ medium squash or pumpkin, cut into thick round slices to resemble a circle

Few sprigs of fresh parsley for garnish

Sea salt

Preheat oven to 190°C/375°F. Meanwhile prepare the onion gravy by heating a large saucepan with some olive oil. Add the onions, a pinch of sea salt and the bay leaves. Sauté uncovered for 10 minutes on a medium flame. Then cover the pan, lower the heat and slowly simmer for at least 45 minutes. The longer it cooks the sweeter it will be. At the end of cooking, add a small amount of white miso (mixed in a small amount of water) and mirin to taste. Dilute some kuzu with a very small amount of cold water, mix well and add to the onions. Stir for a few minutes until translucent and thicker in consistency.

While the gravy is simmering, place the pumpkin slices on an oven tray. Add a few drops of olive oil and a pinch of sea salt on each slice. Cover with foil and bake in the preheated oven for 45 minutes or until the slices are soft. Remove and serve with the onion sauce placed in the center of the pumpkin, and garnish with parsley.

Sweet and Sour Red Cabbage – German Style

1 tbsp sesame oil

2 onions, sliced into thin half moons

2 small apples, peeled, cored and thinly sliced

1 medium red cabbage, thinly sliced

1 tsp salt

Bay leaves (optional)

Small amount of water

Brown rice vinegar

Umeboshi vinegar

Place the oil into a pot and slowly heat and sauté the onions. Add the apples next, then the red cabbage, salt and bay leaves. You may need to add a small amount of water to keep it from burning. Cover the pot, bring to a boil and then turn the heat down. Simmer for approximately 1 hour and season with rice vinegar and umeboshi vinegar to taste. Simmer a little longer until all the flavors are mingled and the cabbage is very soft. Serve hot.

Onion Ring Tempura with Noodles and Broth

Broth

1 pack soba or udon noodles

1 strip of kombu

1½ liters (2½ pints) of water

2 onions, cut into half moons

1 carrot, cut into matchsticks

Tamari and mirin

1–2 tsp juice squeezed from grated fresh ginger

Tempura

½ cup plain flour

½ cup rice flour

3 tbsp arrowroot powder

1 tsp roasted sesame seeds

Cold sparkling water

Organic sunflower frying oil for deep frying

1 medium onion, thinly sliced and separated into rings

Tamari or shoyu

Fresh watercress for garnish

Pinch of sea salt

Cook the noodles according to the packet, rinse and drain. Boil 1½ liters (2½ pints) of water with the kombu strip for 20 minutes. Add the onions and simmer uncovered for 10 minutes. Add the carrots and simmer 5 minutes. Season with tamari and mirin and add the grated ginger juice.

To make the onion ring tempura, combine the flour, arrowroot, salt and sesame seeds, add some cold sparkling water and mix thoroughly into a smooth batter. Place in the refrigerator for one hour.

Heat a frying pan with enough oil for deep frying. Submerge each onion ring into the batter and deep fry for 2–3 minutes until lightly golden and very crisp. Remove each ring and drain on a paper towel.

To serve, fill individual bowls with the cooked noodles and cover with the broth. Top with the tempura onion rings, garnished with watercress. Pour some shoyu or tamari into small individual bowls and serve on the side as a dipping sauce.

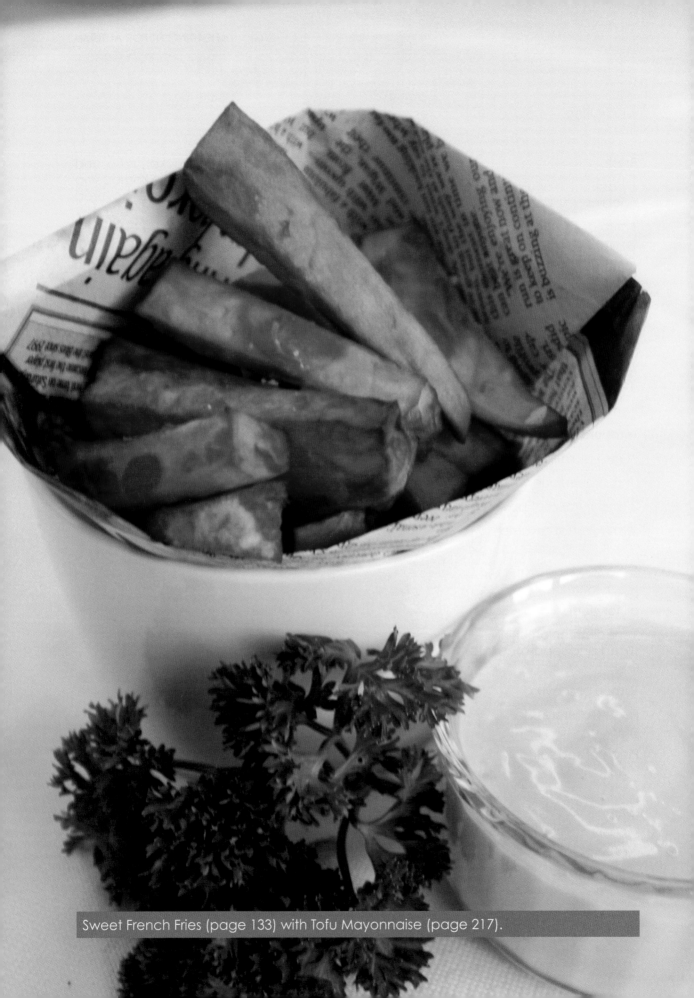

Sweet French Fries (page 133) with Tofu Mayonnaise (page 217).

Beet Fry

1 medium beet, unpeeled

1 medium parsnip, peeled and grated

¼ tsp dried thyme, crumbled

3 tbsp olive oil

1 tbsp finely chopped scallion

Fresh thyme sprigs

Preheat oven to 180°C/350°F. Place the beet in a small baking pan and bake until tender – about 1 hour. Remove from the oven and allow to cool, then grate and combine with the parsnip and crumbled thyme. Lightly sauté the scallion in a tablespoon of olive oil, then add the beet and parsnip mixture and cook for about three minutes. Add the remaining two tablespoons of olive oil and cook over a low heat, stirring continuously for 10 minutes. Sprinkle with thyme sprigs and serve.

Grain Dishes

Millet Croquettes

½ cup carrots, cut into matchsticks

2 cups cooked millet

½ cup minced parsley

Wholewheat pastry flour

Dry wheat flour

Sunflower oil

Pinch of sea salt

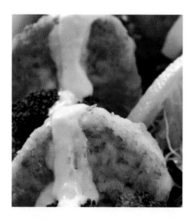

Boil the carrots with a pinch of sea salt in about half an inch of water for 2 to 3 minutes or until soft. Save the water for a sauce. Strain the carrots and mix them together with the cooked millet and minced parsley. Make into round balls or oval shapes. If too dry, add a little wholewheat pastry flour with a little water to keep the shape. If too wet, roll the ball in dry wheat flour. After shaping, deep fry the balls in hot sunflower oil. Cook the balls until they are golden brown and crunchy. Serve with one of the sauces on pages 181–183.

Buckwheat

Buckwheat is an excellent alternative to millet for preparing croquettes. You can also mince and boil celery, or rinse and boil arame, to add to the grains when making the croquettes. Leftover beans can also be cooked this way – lentils and chickpeas are the best.

Squash Risotto

1 tbsp olive oil

1 clove garlic, minced

1 onion, finely diced

2 cups squash, peeled and cut into small cubes

1 tsp marjoram

4 cups cooked brown rice

1.5 liters (2½ pints) vegetable stock or bouillon

Pepper (if desired)

1 tbsp non-dairy cream

Parsley

Sea salt

Heat the olive oil in a heavy-bottomed pan and add the garlic for a moment before adding the onions. Fry on a low-medium heat until the onions are translucent. Add the squash and marjoram and a pinch of salt, and fry for 5 minutes. Cover with one centimeter (half an inch) of water and cook until the squash is soft. Add the rice and then, bit by bit, add hot stock, each time waiting until it is absorbed by the rice. Continue until the rice becomes creamy – this should take about 10 minutes. Finish with pepper (optional), non-dairy cream and parsley.

Mushroom Soba Noodles Topped with Shredded Nori

⅓ cup shitake mushrooms

3 large onions, chopped

1 clove garlic, crushed

1 red pepper de-seeded and thinly sliced

2 tsp basil

2 tsp thyme

½ tsp black pepper

2 tbsp tamari

Handful of shredded nori

1 cup water

1 block tofu

2 tbsp kuzu or arrowroot powder

1 tsp sea salt

1 packet (250 g/9 oz) soba noodles

1 bunch greens (steamed)

1 cup almonds

Soak the shitake mushrooms for 15 minutes or more until soft, then remove the stalk and slice them. Stir fry the onions with the garlic, red pepper, herbs, black pepper and tamari, and then add the mushrooms. When the onions are brown, add half a cup of water and simmer for 15 minutes. Dry roast the almonds and crush them. Crumble the tofu by hand and add to the mushroom mixture. Let it simmer for another five minutes, then stir in kuzu or arrowroot dissolved in a little water to thicken. Seasoning the mushroom sauce with sea salt.

Cook and drain the soba noodles, refresh in cold water and serve with the steamed greens and the mushroom sauce on top. Decorate with the crushed almonds and top with shredded nori.

Rice Croquettes

1 bottle organic sunflower oil for frying

2 cups brown sushi rice

½ cup oat flakes

Recipe One

1 tbsp shoyu

½ carrot, grated

½ leek, finely chopped

Recipe Two

2 tbsp shoyu

1 tbsp lemon zest

1 tsp umeboshi paste

Dipping Sauce

2 tbsp shoyu

4 tbsp water

Freshly grated ginger juice (optional)

Combine the rice and oat flakes. Mix in the shoyu, grated carrot and chopped leek for recipe one, or the shoyu, lemon zest and umeboshi purée for recipe two. Form into small balls, which need to be firm; otherwise they will fall apart when you cook them. Heat the oil. You can usually cook three or four croquettes at a time, depending on the size of the pan. Fry the rice balls until crisp and lightly browned.

For the dipping sauce, mix the shoyu and water together and serve with the croquettes. If you prefer, add a little freshly grated ginger juice to the dipping sauce.

Quinoa with Roasted Butternut Squash, Cranberries and Pecans

½ cup quinoa, washed and drained

½ cup corn

1½ cups water

1 small/medium butternut squash, peeled and diced

½ cup fresh or frozen cranberries, halved or chopped as you prefer

½ medium red onion, finely diced

1 clove of garlic, minced

Olive oil

1–2 tsp pure maple syrup

½ cup chopped pecans

2 tbsp fresh chopped parsley

Sprinkle of cumin or ginger

Sea salt

Ground pepper

Fruity extra virgin olive oil

Place the quinoa, corn, water and a pinch of sea salt in a pan over medium-high heat. Bring to a boil then reduce the heat to medium-low and cook until all the water has been absorbed – about 10 minutes. Meanwhile, preheat oven to 190°C/375°F.

Place the butternut squash, cranberries, onion and garlic in a medium roasting pan and drizzle with a little olive oil, to coat. Add maple syrup – not too much, and sprinkle with sea salt. Toss everything together. Roast in the top half of the oven until the squash is tender – about 15 to 20 minutes. Remove the pan and set aside.

Heat a large dry pan and lightly toast the pecans briefly, till fragrant. Add in the cooked quinoa and the butternut mixture. Add the following to taste: parsley, cumin or ginger, sea salt and ground pepper. Drizzle the quinoa mixture with some fruity extra virgin olive oil and toss to coat. Taste and adjust seasonings. Heat through gently and serve.

Beans and Bean Products

French Green Lentil and Vegetable Roast

5 shitake mushrooms

2 tbsp olive oil

1 small onion, diced

1 carrot, peeled and diced

2 stalks celery, diced

2 cloves garlic, crushed

2 sprigs thyme, taken off the stalks

½ cup dry French green lentils

2 tbsp shoyu

Small piece of kombu

2 tsp brown rice miso

½ cup brown breadcrumbs

¼ cup ground almonds, toasted

3 tbsp sesame seeds, toasted

Soak the shitake in warm water for about 10 minutes until soft. Remove and discard the stalks and then finely chop the mushrooms. Reserve the soaking liquid. Heat the oil in a pan and fry the onion, carrot and celery for 5 minutes. Add the garlic and thyme, and fry for a further 2 minutes. Add the lentils, shoyu, followed by the kombu and shitake soaking liquid. Let the lentils boil rapidly for 10 minutes and then simmer for a further 40 minutes or until the lentils are soft. Stir the pot every now and then.

Preheat the oven to 190°C/375°F. Take the kombu out of the lentil pot and put in a blender with half the lentil mix and the miso, blend until smooth and then put back into the lentil pot. Stir in the rest of the ingredients and a good twist of black pepper until they are evenly mixed. Pour the mixture into an oiled loaf pan and bake for 1 hour. When it is ready, remove from the oven and allow to rest for a couple of minutes. Use a palette knife to loosen the edges and then turn out onto a serving dish. Serve with either Onion Gravy (see page 168) or Rich Gravy (see page 183).

Glazed Tempeh

¼ cup fresh orange juice

¼ cup balsamic vinegar

1 tbsp sesame oil

1 tsp soy sauce

2 cloves fresh garlic, crushed

1 tbsp finely minced fresh basil or 1 tsp dried basil

1 tbsp finely minced fresh flat-leaf parsley or 1 tsp dried parsley

1 pack tempeh, cut into slices

2 bunches spring greens, rinsed, stems trimmed and sliced

2 tbsp fresh lemon juice

Sea salt

Combine the orange juice, vinegar, oil, soy sauce, garlic, basil and parsley in a pan over a medium heat. When the mixture is hot, arrange the tempeh slices in the mixture and cook until browned – about 4 minutes. Turn and brown on the other side – about 4 minutes more. While the tempeh braises, place about a centimeter (half an inch) of water and a pinch of sea salt in the bottom of a saucepan and bring to a boil. Add the greens and steam until they are just wilted and bright green – about 3 minutes. Arrange the steamed greens on a plate and place the tempeh slices on top. Sprinkle with lemon juice.

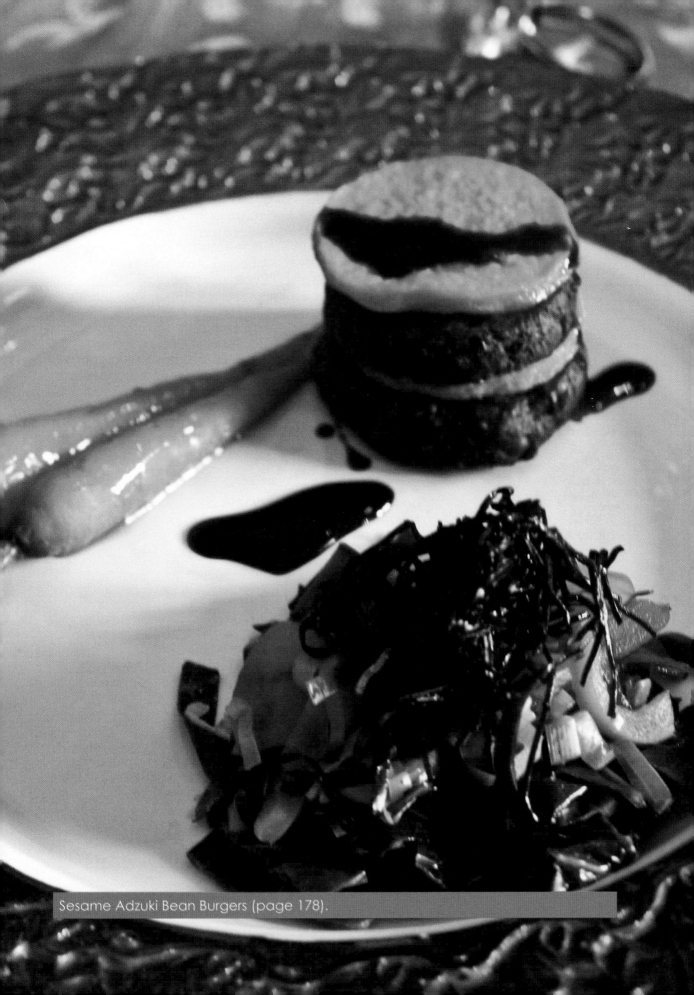

Sesame Adzuki Bean Burgers (page 178).

Sesame Adzuki Bean Burger

Makes 6–7 patties.

1 tbsp sesame oil

½ cup of diced onion

3 stalks celery, diced

2 cloves garlic, minced

1 tbsp fresh ginger, minced

½ red bell pepper, diced

3 cups stemmed, chopped kale

2 ⅔ cup cooked and drained adzuki beans, divided

3 tbsp tahini

2 tbsp water, or as needed

¼ cup sesame seeds (optional)

Preheat oven to 190°C/375°F and lightly oil a baking sheet. Heat the oil in a large pan over a medium heat and add the onion, celery, garlic and ginger. Cook, stirring occasionally, until the onions are softened and beginning to brown – about 5 minutes. Stir in the bell pepper and kale, and cook, covered, until the kale has wilted – another 5 minutes or so. Remove from the heat.

Meanwhile, purée two cups of the adzuki beans, tahini and water in a food processor. It doesn't have to be completely smooth, but make sure the ingredients are well incorporated. Transfer to a large mixing bowl and stir in the vegetable mixture and remaining two-thirds of a cup of whole adzuki beans. Sprinkle sesame seeds on a large plate, if using. Using wet hands, scoop out about a half to three-quarters of a cup of the mixture and form into a ball. Flatten slightly and press into the sesame seeds, if using, then transfer to a baking sheet. Repeat with the remaining mixture. Bake at for 20 minutes, turning once halfway through, or until a slight crust has formed. Meanwhile, slice the neck of a butternut squash into equal sizes, drizzle with olive oil and bake in the oven for 15–20 minutes. Serve the burgers topped with the baked pumpkin slices.

Mixed Mushroom Gravy

2 tbsp olive oil

125 g (4 oz) button mushrooms

125 g (4 oz) fresh shitake mushrooms, sliced

2 tbsp all-purpose flour

1 cup unflavored rice milk

1 cup Dashi Stock (see page 69)

½ tsp salt

½ tsp white pepper (optional)

Browning the flour helps give this gravy a rich, nutty flavor. Heat one tablespoon of olive oil in a saucepan over a medium heat. Add all the mushrooms and sauté for 5 minutes. Stir in the flour and remaining one tablespoon of oil. Reduce the heat to low and cook for 10 minutes, or until the flour begins to brown, whisking constantly. Whisk in the rice milk, Dashi Stock, salt and white pepper. Simmer for 15 minutes, or until thickened, whisking often.

Smothered Seitan Medallions in Mixed Mushroom Gravy

1 pack seitan, cut into medallions

5 tbsp arrowroot powder

1 cup plus 2 tbsp olive oil, divided

1 large onion, thinly sliced (2 cups)

5 cloves garlic, minced (2 tbsp)

2 cups Mixed Mushroom Gravy (see page 178)

2 cups miso bouillon stock

1 cup finely chopped green cabbage

¼ cup thinly sliced scallions

2 tbsp chopped parsley

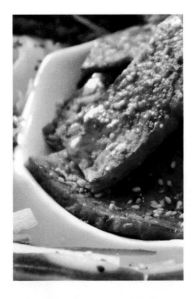

Coat the seitan pieces with arrowroot and heat half a cup of oil in a pan over a medium-high heat. Fry half of seitan in oil for 3 minutes per side. Transfer to a paper-towel-lined plate. Discard the oil, wipe out the pan, and repeat with half a cup of oil and the remaining seitan. Discard the oil. Add the remaining two tablespoons of oil and onion to the hot pan. Increase the heat to high and sauté for 3 minutes. Reduce the heat to medium and sauté 10 minutes more. Add the garlic and sauté for 3 minutes. Stir in the mushroom gravy, miso stock and seitan. Cover and simmer for 30 minutes. Add the cabbage and cook for 3 minutes. Stir in the scallions and parsley.

Millet and Tofu Bake with Pressed Chicory, Radish and Cucumber Salad

Pressed Salad

Cucumber, finely diced

Chicory, finely sliced

Radishes, sliced into half moons

1 tsp umeboshi vinegar

Millet and Tofu Bake

1 onion, finely sliced

2 medium carrots, finely sliced into half moons

½ pack tofu

½ cup cooked millet

2 tbsp shoyu

1 tbsp brown rice vinegar

Sesame oil

Black toasted sesame seeds

Combine the pressed salad ingredients together in a salad press and add a teaspoon of umeboshi vinegar. Close and press the salad for 1 hour.

Sauté the onions and carrots in sesame oil for about 10 minutes until soft. Scramble the tofu with your hands into a bowl and add the onions, carrots and millet. Add the shoyu and brown rice vinegar. Mix together and transfer to an ovenproof dish. Bake for 20 minutes on a medium heat.

Serve the tofu bake in a small bowl, garnished with the pressed salad, and sprinkle with black toasted sesame seeds.

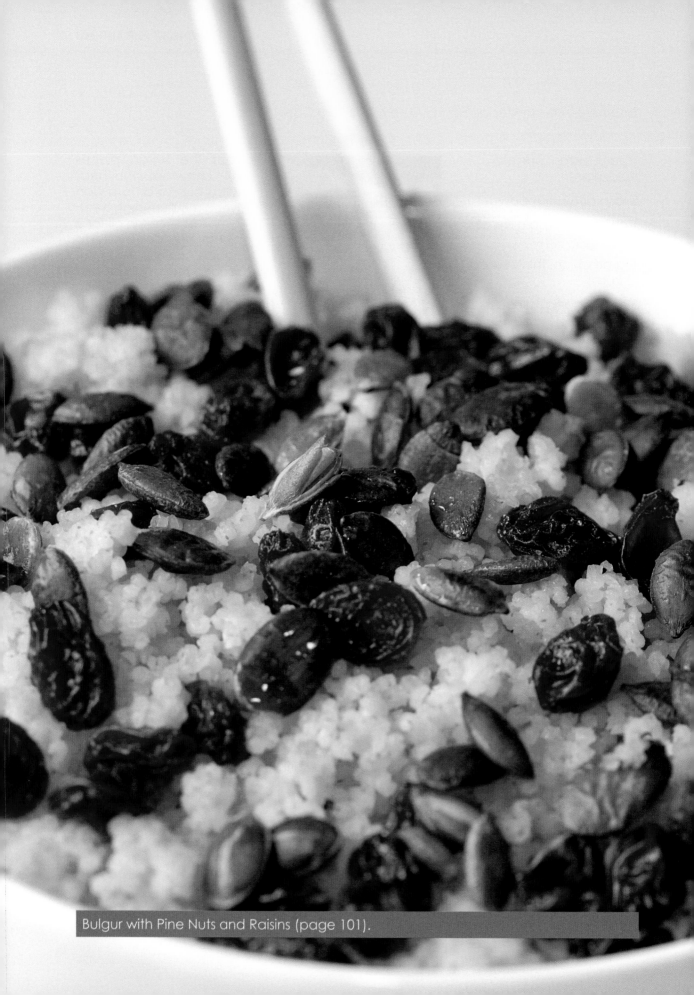

Bulgur with Pine Nuts and Raisins (page 101).

Sauces, Salads and Side Dishes

Cooking with seaweed (sea vegetables)

Sea vegetables are enriched with all the minerals that support life, and in fact contain twenty times more minerals than land vegetables – minerals such as calcium, iron, potassium, iodine and magnesium, not to mention the trace minerals so necessary for body functions. This is an incredible food, packed with nutrition. Sea plants do not absorb pollution from the ocean in the same way that fish do and have a great ability to remove radioactive and metallic poisons from the body, especially from the kidneys. These vegetables are high in vitamins A, B, C, D, E and K, and can help the body dissolve fat in and around the various organ systems of the body. They also contain chlorophyll, which aids in the production of hemoglobin, strengthening red blood cells.

Hijiki Sauté

2 tsp light sesame oil

1 cup hijiki, soaked for about 10 minutes until tender, then drained

1–2 tbsp mirin

1 onion, thinly sliced

1 carrot, cut into matchsticks

Spring or filtered water

Soy sauce (tamari or shoyu)

Toasted sesame seeds

Heat the sesame oil in a pan over a medium heat. Add the hijiki and cook, stirring constantly for about 5 minutes. Add the mirin and enough water to half cover and simmer over a low heat for 20 minutes. Add the onion and carrot, season lightly with soy sauce, cover and simmer for 10 minutes. Remove the cover and allow to cook until any remaining liquid has been absorbed. Transfer to a bowl and serve with toasted sesame seeds.

Carrot and Onion Sauce

2 tbsp extra virgin olive oil

1 clove garlic, minced

½ cup carrots, diced

1 onion, finely chopped

3 tbsp organic unbleached white flour

3 tbsp shoyu

1 cup water

½ tsp sea salt

½ cup cauliflower, small florets

1 cup green peas, fresh or frozen

2 tsp fresh chives, finely chopped, or fresh parsley, for garnish

Heat the oil in a saucepan. Sauté the garlic, carrots and onions for 3 minutes. Add flour and stir constantly until the vegetables are coated with the flour. Combine the shoyu and water. Slowly add to the pan, stirring or whisking constantly to prevent lumping. Simmer until thick. Add sea salt, cauliflower and pepper to taste. Cover and simmer on a low heat for 5 to 7 minutes or until the onions and cauliflower are tender. Add the peas, then cover and simmer for another 3 minutes. Turn off the flame, mix in the chives and season with black pepper. Serve as a side dish or as a sauce over any organic pasta or cooked organic grain.

Rich Gravy

3 shitake mushrooms

1 large onion, thinly sliced

1 tsp sesame oil

2 tbsp tahini

2 tbsp soy sauce

5 tsp kuzu

1 tbsp mirin

Rinse the mushrooms and soak in three cups of water for ½ hour. Drain, reserving the soaking liquid. Cut the mushrooms into slices, discarding the hard tips of the stems. Sauté the onions and mushrooms in the toasted sesame oil for 15 minutes. Add the reserved soaking water, cover and bring to a boil. Mix together the tahini and soy sauce and gently stir into the onions and mushrooms. Lower the heat and simmer for 5 minutes. Completely dissolve the kuzu in half a cup of cool water. Turn the heat to high and add the kuzu, stirring constantly until the kuzu begins to brown. Lower the heat, stir in the mirin and simmer for 5 minutes.

Pressed Daikon Salad

1 cup finely sliced daikon

2 cups finely sliced cucumber

1 tbsp finely minced parsley

2 tbsp toasted sesame seeds

1 tbsp umeboshi vinegar

¼ granny smith apple, grated

Shoyu

Pinch of sea salt

Place the daikon, cucumber and parsley in a bowl and mix with the sea salt. Transfer to a pickle press and press for 30 minutes. Grind the sesame seeds to a fine powder in a suribachi. Add the umeboshi and one drop of shoyu to the seeds and mix. Open the press and remove any excess water. Add the seeds and grated apple and mix through the vegetables.

Desserts

Sweet Winter Squash and Pear Dessert

½ Hokkaido or other sweet winter squash, peeled and cut into large chunks

4 pears, peeled and cut into large chunks

Zest of 1 orange

1 vanilla pod

½ tsp cinnamon powder

Pinch of sea salt

Non-dairy whipped cream

Black sesame seeds

Place the winter squash and pears in a heavy-based pan and cover the bottom of the pan with water. Bring to a boil and then cook on a very low heat until the squash and pears are soft. Purée with a hand blender and then add the orange zest, vanilla pod and cinnamon powder. Stir the mixture then serve in individual glass bowls, topped with some non-dairy whipped cream, and sprinkle with black sesame seeds.

Apricot Cream

1 cup dried apricots

½ cup water

1 cup apple juice

2 medium apples, peeled and cubed

½ tsp cinnamon powder

1 tbsp almond or hazelnut butter

Roasted almonds, chopped

Pinch of sea salt

Put the apricots in a small pot and cover with water, apple juice and salt. Bring to a boil and simmer for 15 minutes. Add the apples and cinnamon and more liquid if needed. Cook until the apples are soft and the liquid has been absorbed. Transfer to a blender and purée with the almond or hazelnut butter until smooth. Serve decorated with Tofu and Vanilla Whip (see page 153) and roasted chopped almonds.

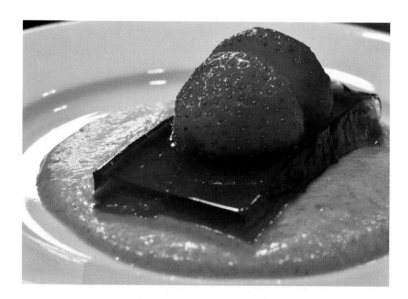

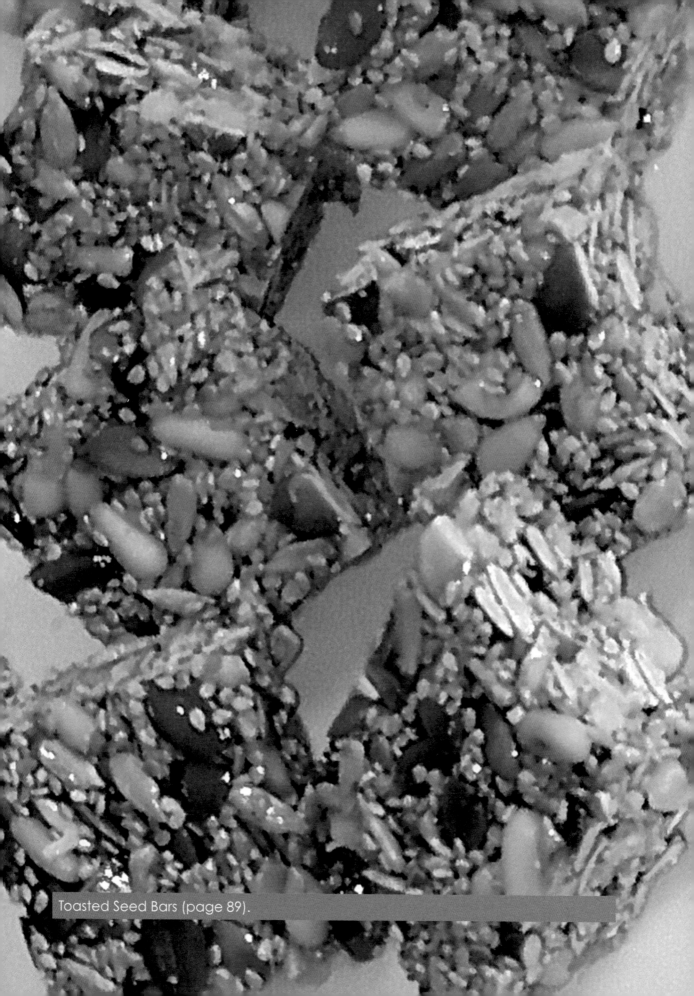

Toasted Seed Bars (page 89).

Apple Crisp

Topping

½ cup wholewheat flour

1½ cups rolled oats

2 tbsp corn oil

¼ cup brown rice syrup

½ cup sunflower seeds

2 tbsp chopped walnuts

⅛ tsp sea salt

½ tsp cinnamon powder

Filling

8–10 apples, peeled and sliced

½ cup raisins

1 heaping tsp kuzu

⅔ cup apple juice

⅓ cup water

½ tsp vanilla

Place the flour and oats in a bowl. Heat the oil and rice syrup until mixed, then stir into the flour and oats. Add the seeds, nuts, salt and cinnamon and set aside.

Preheat oven to 190°C/375°F. Spread the apples and raisins in a 22×30 cm (9×12–inch) baking dish. Dissolve the kuzu in the juice and water, heat and stir until thick. Remove from the heat and stir in the vanilla. Pour over the fruit and spoon on the topping. Bake at 190°C/375°F for 45 minutes until bubbly. Serve warm or chilled, with non-dairy whipped cream if desired.

Apple Walnut Muffins

1 cup whole spelt flour

1 cup white spelt flour

3 tsp baking powder

½ tsp baking soda

1 tsp cinnamon

½ cup chopped walnuts

2 apples, peeled and chopped

1 cup rice or soy milk

1 cup rice syrup

1 tsp vanilla essence

½ cup baking oil

Preheat oven to 155°C/310°F. Mix all the dry ingredients together in a bowl. Add the walnuts and apples. In a jug or measuring cup blend the wet ingredients and add to the dry mixture, stirring in gently. Oil a muffin tray or use muffin cases, add a good tablespoon of the mixture to each and bake for 30 minutes.

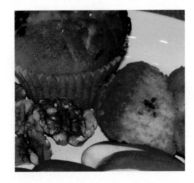

Chapter 10

HALE AND HEARTY IN WINTER

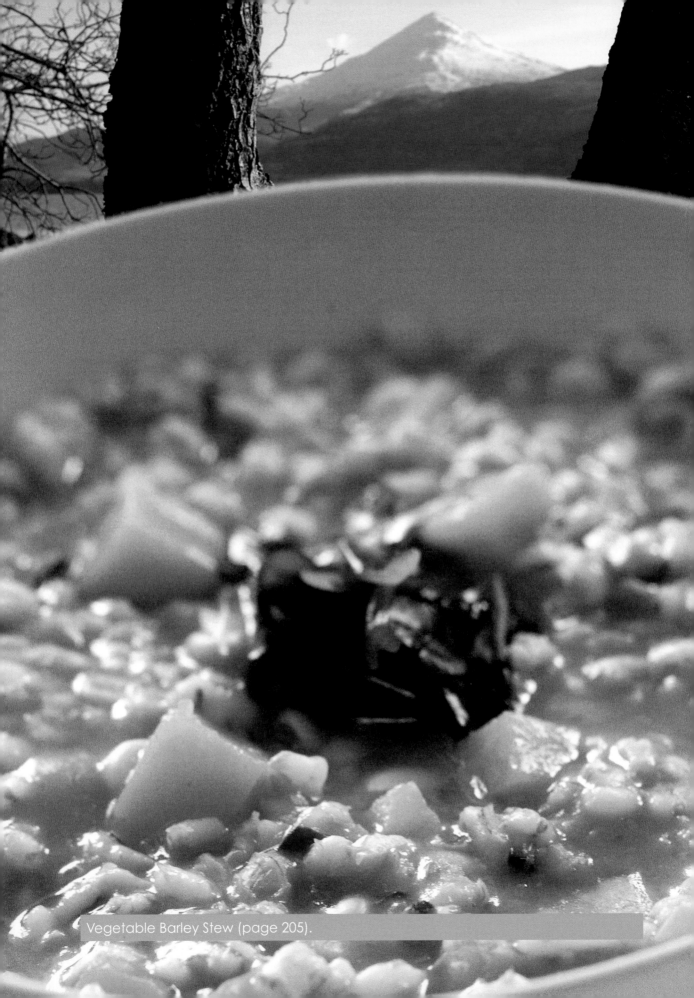

Vegetable Barley Stew (page 205).

Winter was such a fun time for my family. It was so cold with lots of snow before the climate started to change and warm up. There was no such thing as a greenhouse effect then, I guess. Coming from a large family of six girls and one boy, we had the most incredible household, filled with love, fun and laughter. There were seven single beds – one for each of us. On the cold winter nights, when mum and dad were asleep, we would all sneak in bed beside each other and huddle up as we watched the icicles form on the windowpanes (there wasn't any central heating in those days). The coal fire was always roaring when we rose early in the morning to eat our porridge and line up (by age, youngest first) for a spoonful of Delrosa rose hip syrup before marching off to school. Talk about the von Trapps – we had our very own *Sound of Music* theme happening.

Winter is when the life energy of the earth settles deep within the soil. It is the time of moving within, both socially and physically. The energy of the body wants to move deeper and we have a tendency to conserve energy needed for warmth. We move indoors more and socialize with family and friends. There is a drift towards contemplation and reflection on the past seasons and making plans for the future.

General Considerations

As we approach the year-end and look forward to the New Year, the Northern and Southern hemispheres are experiencing seasons that are literally poles apart. Winter solstice is the day of the year (normally December 21) when the sun is farthest south. It marks the first day of the season of winter and the shortest day of the year, in the sense that the length of time elapsed between sunrise and sunset on this particular day is the minimum for the year.

Winter is ruled by the WATER element, which is associated with the kidneys, bladder and adrenal glands. It is a time when nature is silent and still, and at rest. In order to rejuvenate the body and the mind, we also need rest and warmth. The kidneys are of paramount importance to overall physical health and are considered to be the most vulnerable organs at this time of year.

Exercises that help to generate heat and energy in the kidneys, such as certain Pilates and Yoga postures, are extremely beneficial. The kidney energy is also depleted in the winter by long hours of work, excessive exercise or punishing fitness regimes. Little rest, lack of sleep and eating cooling foods are inappropriate for this time of year. If we dampen the warmth of the body in the winter months we are susceptible to colds and fevers.

Health is greatly enhanced by going to bed earlier in the winter and eating good, wholesome hot foods, such as whole grains, legumes, stews, soups and warming dinners. This is the season to give yourself permission for a lie in and to encourage yourself to go to bed early. If we take care of our energy in winter and guard against energy expenditure by cultivating quietness and contemplation, we will find ourselves feeling refreshed and healthy in spring.

The body heals and balances itself more quickly when we are still and deeply relaxed. From a place of stillness and deep reflection, we are able to flow with life and change our attitudes, perceptions and life habits with less resistance and personal drama. Nurturing the WATER element is the best way to ensure a long life.

Something Like Winter

The cooking and food choices outlined for winter are all about warming the body and strengthening the WATER element. If a person is living on a diet all year round that is better suited to hot climates or warm months, they may suffer damage to the kidneys, adrenal glands or sexual organs. The lower areas of the body or kidneys may feel cold, sexual energy may diminish or there may be a weakness in the bones. How many times have you heard someone say that they were chilled to the bone? Cooking for winter can be helpful when the body is locked into a cold condition.

Special Drinks and Home Remedies

Black Soybean Tea

Recommended for bone and joint disorders or kidney and bladder problems.

1 cup black soybeans

5 cm (2 inch) strip kombu, soaked and finely chopped

4 cups water

Place the soybeans in a pot with the kombu. Add the water and bring to a boil. Lower the flame and simmer for 30 to 45 minutes. Strain the beans and drink this slightly sweet liquid while hot. You may continue cooking the beans longer until soft and edible for regular consumption.

Adzuki Bean Tea

A great drink for strengthening the kidney, bladder or adrenals.

1 cup adzuki beans

5 cm (2 inch) strip kombu

4 cups water

Place the adzuki beans in

a pot with the kombu seaweed and soak for 4 hours or overnight. Finely chop the kombu, add the water and bring to a boil. Lower the flame, cover and simmer for approximately 20–30 minutes. Strain out the beans and drink the liquid while hot. You may continue cooking the beans longer with additional water, until soft and edible.

Kidney Drink

Rejuvenates, detoxes and strengthens the kidney function.

Soaked adzuki beans

Shredded dried daikon

Dried shitake mushrooms

Kombu

Water

Prepare this special drink by combining one part each of adzuki beans, daikon, shitake mushrooms and kombu. Add five times as much water, boil, and then simmer for about 25 minutes. Take one cup of this tea every day for 10 days.

Shoyu Bancha Tea

This drink is good for strengthening the blood if an overly acidic condition exists, relieving fatigue, alleviating headaches due to overconsumption of simple sugars and/or fruit juice, and stimulating good blood circulation.

1 tsp shoyu

Bancha twig or bancha stem tea

Place the shoyu in a teacup and pour in hot bancha tea that has been made a little stronger than usual. Stir well and drink hot.

Ginger Compress

A ginger compress is an amazing restorative for all that ails you.

The purpose of a hot ginger compress is to dissolve stagnation, mucus and tension, melt blockages and stimulate circulation and energy flow. This is a wonderful treatment for injuries to the body, especially the back, and is particularly good for moving stagnated chi in the kidneys and the lungs. It also helps heal skin complaints. The heat activity of the compress stimulates the blood and tissue circulation in the area being treated, which then facilitates the excretion of the dispersed toxins. It is effective in dissolving hardened accumulations of fats, proteins or minerals, including kidney stones, gall bladder stones, cysts and benign tumors such as uterine fibroids.

Many types of acute or chronic pain can be relieved, such as rheumatism, arthritis, backaches, cramps, kidney stone attacks, toothaches, stiff neck and similar problems. A ginger compress can speed up the improvement from a variety of inflammatory conditions, such as bronchitis, prostate infection, and bladder and intestinal inflammations (but never appendicitis). It is effective in relieving congestive conditions like asthma. If tissues have been damaged, a ginger compress can speed up the regeneration of the damaged area. It is a wonderful remedy for dispelling muscle tension.

Bring a large pot of water to a boil. Meanwhile, grate enough ginger root to equal the size of a golf ball. When the water comes to a boil, reduce the heat to low, and place the ginger into a cotton handkerchief and tie with string or secure with an elastic band. The water at this point should be just below boiling point. Place the ball into the pot and allow it to soak in the water without boiling for about 5 minutes.

Place a facecloth into the ginger water, wring out and apply to the desired area on the body. Cover with a hand towel to hold in the heat. Change the facecloth every 2 to 3 minutes as it starts to cool off. This can be done by using two cloths and alternating them so that the skin does not cool off between applications. Continue the applications for about 15 to 20 minutes.

The tissues of the walls of the intestine begin to receive clean, revitalized blood (provided we have also changed our way of eating, and it has to emphasized that the ginger compress is a waste of time if we do not). The intestines become revitalized, leading to regeneration of the tissues and restoration of their proper, harmonious function.

As a result of doing the treatment, mucus deposits are gradually dissolved and toxins are flushed into the bloodstream. The body may show signs of detoxification or may show no overt signs of cleansing other than passive weight loss, increased urination and bowel movement, and some fatigue. If accompanied by a healthy appetite, normal sleep patterns, good vitality and no nausea, these signs indicate the healing process is going well.

The compress should be done twice a week. For psoriasis, place the hot towels starting from the sternum down to the navel so as to cover the whole intestinal tract. *Never* apply a ginger compress when a high fever is present. Because the compresses are very contractive (yang), they are hot applications and therefore should not be used on a dense area of the body such as the brain.

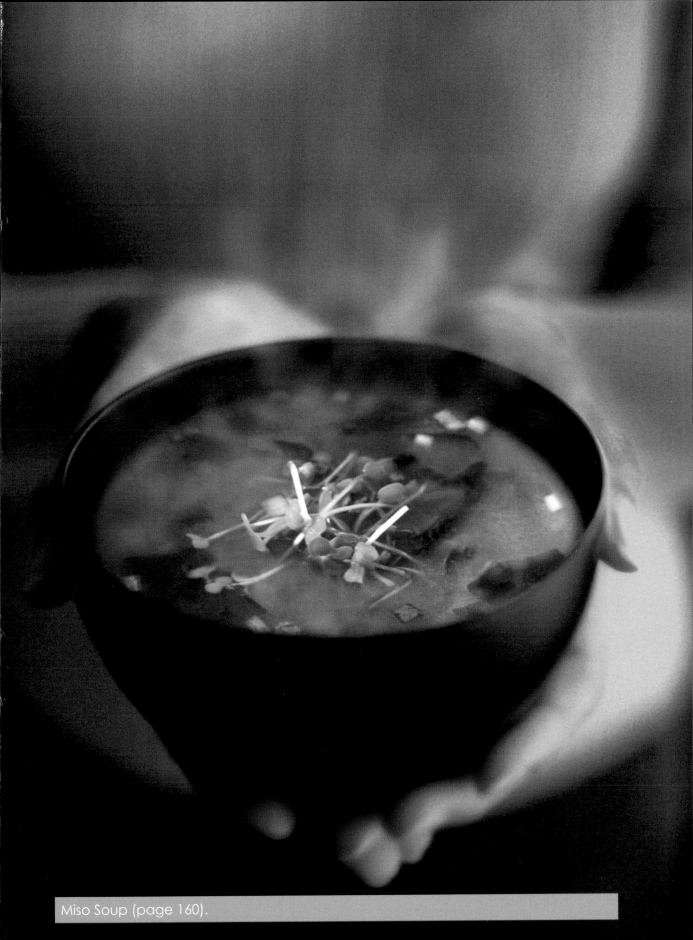

Miso Soup (page 160).

Recipes for Winter

(Each recipe yields 4 servings)

Soups

Creamy Zucchini and Leek Soup

2 leeks, sliced in half lengthwise and cut into small pieces

1–2 strips of wakame, rinsed and cut into pieces

2 zucchini, sliced

2 cups water

White miso

Olive oil

Dried basil

Pinch of sea salt

Heat a pot with a small amount of oil and add the leeks and a pinch of salt. Sauté uncovered for 5–6 minutes. Add the rinsed wakame, zucchini, dried basil and two cups of water. Cover and cook on a medium flame for 15–20 minutes. Blend to a smooth consistency, adjusting the liquid if necessary. Add some white miso to taste.

Vegetable Bisque Soup with Fresh Basil

1 tsp avocado oil

½ red onion, diced

1 carrot, diced

1 stalk celery, diced

1 parsnip, diced

1 cup butternut squash

1 cup diced green cabbage

1 small sweet potato, diced

4 cups Dashi Stock (see page 69) or filtered water

1 bay leaf

2 tsp sweet white miso

Scant pinch of fresh nutmeg

2 stalks fresh basil, leaves removed and shredded

Sea salt

Heat the oil in a soup pot over a medium heat. Add the onion and a pinch of salt and sauté until translucent – about 3 minutes. Stir in the carrot and a pinch of salt, and sauté for 1 minute. Add the celery, parsnip, squash, cabbage and sweet potato, followed each time by a pinch of salt and sautéing for one minute before adding the next ingredient. Add water or Dashi Stock and a bay leaf. Bring to a boil, cover and reduce the heat to low and cook until the vegetables are tender – about 30 minutes. Remove the bay leaf and discard. Use a hand blender and purée the soup until smooth. Remove a small amount of soup and stir in the miso until dissolved. Stir the miso mixture and nutmeg into the soup and simmer for 3 to 4 minutes. Serve garnished with basil.

Dulse Onion Soup

Dulse is a super sea vegetable and like other seaweed is low in calories but offers an abundance of vitamins and minerals.

1 tsp sesame oil

1 medium onion, diced

½ cup dried dulse

4 cups spring water or Dashi Stock (see page 69)

½ cup rolled oats

2 tbsp white miso

1 tbsp parsley, finely chopped

Heat a large saucepan over a medium heat, add the oil and cook the onion for 2 to 3 minutes. Rinse the dulse under cold water and cut into small pieces, or if using dulse flakes just add to the saucepan. Add the water or Dashi Stock and the oats and bring everything to a boil. Reduce the heat to low, cover and simmer for 15 minutes. Dilute the miso using a small amount of the soup broth. Stir the miso into the broth and cook for 3 to 4 minutes more. Serve garnished with parsley.

French Lentil and Vegetable Soup

1 tbsp extra virgin olive oil

2 cloves fresh garlic, finely minced

½ red onion, diced

2 stalks celery, diced

1 medium carrot, diced

1 cup French green lentils, rinsed

1 cup canned (organic) diced tomatoes

4 cups spring water or Dashi Stock (see page 69)

1 bay leaf

2 stalks flat-leaf parsley, coarsely minced, for garnish

Sea salt

Place the oil, garlic and onion in a medium pot over a medium heat. When the onion begins to sizzle, add a pinch of salt and sauté until translucent – about 3 minutes. Stir in the celery and a pinch of salt and sauté for 1 minute. Stir in carrot and a pinch of salt and sauté for 1 minute. Add the lentils, tomatoes, water (or Dashi Stock) and bay leaf and bring to a boil. Cover, reduce the heat to low and cook until the lentils are soft – about 45 minutes. Season with about one teaspoon of salt and simmer for 5 to 7 minutes more. Remove the bay leaf. Serve with parsley to garnish.

Mushroom and Barley Soup

¼ cup pearl barley, rinsed and drained

6 cups vegetable stock

1 bay leaf

1 tbsp olive oil

1 cup mushrooms, thinly sliced

1 onion, finely chopped

2 carrots, thinly sliced

1 tbsp chopped fresh tarragon

1 tbsp chopped fresh parsley or tarragon for garnish

Bring four cups of the stock to the boil in a small saucepan. Add the bay leaf and, if the stock is unsalted, add a pinch of salt (if required). Stir in the barley, reduce the heat, cover and simmer for 40 minutes.

Heat the oil in a large frying pan over a medium heat. Add the mushrooms and season with salt and pepper. Cook for about 8 minutes until they are golden brown, stirring occasionally at first, then more often after they start to color. Remove the mushrooms from the pan and add the onions and carrots. Cover and cook for about 5 minutes, stirring frequently until the onion is softened. Add the remaining stock and bring to the boil. Stir in the barley with its cooking liquid and add the mushrooms. Discard the bay leaf. Reduce the heat, cover and simmer gently for about 20 minutes, or until the carrots are tender, stirring occasionally. Stir in the tarragon. Taste and adjust the seasoning if necessary. Ladle into warm bowls, garnish with fresh parsley or tarragon and serve.

Turnip Soup

This comforting soup is so subtly flavored that even turnip-haters like it. Baby turnips have a milder taste, but the recipe works just as well with regular turnips.

2 tbsp olive oil

1 kg (2 lb) fresh baby turnips, peeled and diced

1 small onion, diced (1 cup)

2 bay leaves

¼ cup non-dairy milk (optional)

¼ cup celery leaves, chopped

Heat the oil in a large saucepan over a medium heat. Add the turnips and onions, and cook, stirring occasionally, for 15 minutes or until the vegetables are translucent. Add the bay leaves and three cups of water, and season with salt and pepper, if desired. Bring to a boil, reduce the heat to medium-low and cover. Cook for 25 to 30 minutes or until the turnips are very tender. Remove from the heat and take out the bay leaves. Add the milk, if using. Use a blender or food processor to purée the ingredients until smooth. Season with salt and pepper, if desired, and stir in the celery leaves just before serving.

Deep-Fried Mochi in Broth

Deep-fried mochi is delicious in this soup, but also tasty when served with a dip or wrapped in toasted nori strips.

9 pieces mochi

3 tbsp shoyu

2 tbsp mirin

4 cups Dashi Stock (see page 69)

3 scallions, finely chopped

Sunflower oil for deep frying

Finely grated daikon

Heat five centimeters (two inches) of oil in a saucepan to about 170°C/340°F. This is the temperature at which a drop of flour and water batter will sink to the bottom of the pan and immediately rise back up to the surface. Deep fry the mochi until golden brown. Gently place the mochi into individual serving bowls. Warm the Dashi Stock and add the shoyu and mirin. Pour a third of the hot dashi broth over each bowl of mochi and top with the grated daikon and scallions.

Mochi

Mochi is supremely versatile and is generally served as the main ingredient of a meal. Naturally filling and slightly sweet, this rice food is also great on its own as a snack. Mochi is energizing and easy to digest – an excellent food if you are feeling weak. It is eaten regularly in winter for increasing stamina and warmth.

Mochi is really easy to cook. It can be baked, grilled, pan fried or deep fried. When cooked, it puffs up to nearly double its original size, developing a crisp crust outside and a soft, melting interior. Baked or grilled mochi is often eaten with a sweet miso topping. When baked it can be cut into bit-size pieces and added to soups during the last minute of cooking. Pan- or deep-fried mochi doesn't need anything more than a squirt of soy sauce or a dip of soy sauce and fresh ginger. Mochi can be rolled in rice syrup, then coated with ground walnuts and eaten as a dessert.

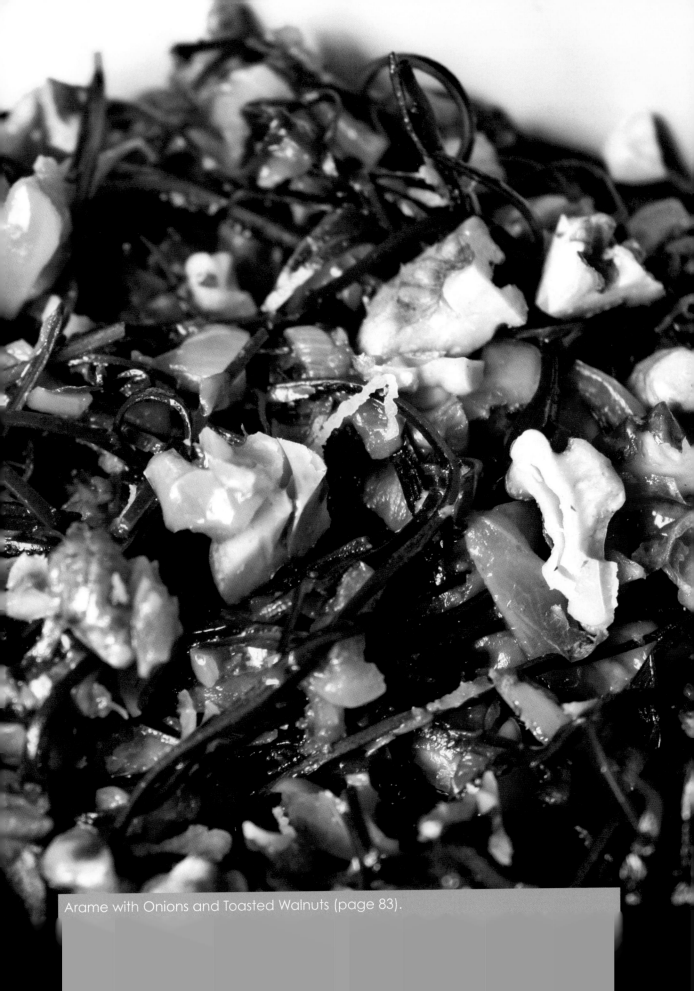

Arame with Onions and Toasted Walnuts (page 83).

Vegetable Dishes

Hearty Greens

Use seasonally available kale, cabbage greens, collards or other hearty greens.

1 bunch greens

Extra virgin olive oil

2 cups chopped onions

Dashi Stock (see page 69)

Sea salt

Wash the greens thoroughly to remove any dust or soil. Slice and remove any hard core. Heat the oil in a heavy-based pan and add the onions and a pinch of sea salt. Allow the onions to sweat over a low heat for about 5 minutes. Add the greens and Dashi Stock and sprinkle another pinch of sea salt over the greens. Cover and cook for 30 minutes. The amount of greens you are cooking will determine the cooking time and how much stock you require. Adjust accordingly.

Kinpira

An incredible dish whose name translates to "sauté and simmer." Kinpira-style cooking is very vitalizing – vegetables are sautéed over a high heat and then simmered to tender perfection. Burdock is used, which is the most strengthening root vegetable known to man.

1 tsp dark or light sesame oil

1 cup burdock, cut into thin matchsticks

1 cup carrot, cut into thin matchsticks

Spring or filtered water

Soy sauce

Heat the sesame oil in a heavy skillet. Sauté the burdock until well coated with oil – about 2 minutes. Spread the burdock evenly over the skillet and top with the carrots. Do not stir. Add just enough water to cover the burdock, cover and cook over a medium-low heat for about 10 minutes. Season lightly with soy sauce and simmer until any liquid that remains has been absorbed – about 10 minutes. Stir well before transferring to a serving platter.

Savory Roasted Vegetables

1 bay leaf

2 cups button mushrooms, brushed clean and left whole

2 cups small Brussels sprouts, trimmed and left whole

2 parsnips cut into large, irregular chunks

2 leeks, rinsed well and cut into 5 cm (2 inch) pieces

2 cups daikon, cut into 2½ cm (1 inch) chunks

Soy sauce

Extra virgin olive oil

Reduced balsamic vinegar

2 tsp fresh lemon juice

Preheat oven to 190°C/375°F. Place the bay leaf on the bottom of a shallow baking dish to help tenderize and sweeten the vegetables. Arrange the vegetable pieces on top, avoiding overlap, and sprinkle lightly with soy sauce and oil, coating the vegetables well. Cover the dish and bake for about 1 hour, until the vegetables are tender. Remove the cover, stir in a light sprinkling of reduced balsamic vinegar and return the dish to the oven to lightly brown the vegetables and turn any remaining liquid into a syrup. Remove the bay leaf and toss gently with lemon juice before serving.

Roasted Broccoli

Broccoli, cut into bite-size pieces

Olive oil

Sea salt

Preheat oven to 200°C/400°F. Place the broccoli on a baking tray with sides. Sprinkle with olive oil and toss with the hands until all the pieces are lightly coated. Repeat the same technique with the sea salt. Place into a hot oven (on the bottom of the oven if not convection). Turn once when the broccoli is greening. Cook until tender.

Baked Cauliflower with Garlic

Cauliflower, cut into medium-size pieces

Whole garlic cloves

Olive oil or light sesame oil

Sea salt

Preheat oven to 180°C/350°F. Place the cauliflower in a baking pan that has a lid. Add whole garlic cloves – as many as you like. Sprinkle a layer of oil on the cauliflower and toss with the hands until all the pieces are lightly coated. Repeat this step with the sea salt. Cover the pot and bake the vegetables in a medium to hot oven until tender.

Roasted Green Beans with Shallots

2 cups green beans

1 shallot, finely chopped

2 tbsp olive oil

Sea salt to taste

Preheat oven to 225°C/425°F. Toss the beans and shallots in oil and arrange on a baking sheet. Sprinkle with sea salt. Roast the vegetables in the oven for 20–25 minutes, or until the beans are blistered and tender.

Maple-Glazed Root Vegetables

Maple-glazed root vegetables, slightly sweet and a charming accompaniment to wintertime suppers, are both satisfying and nourishing.

2 tbsp organic olive oil

3 large carrots, peeled and julienned, ½ cm (¼ inch) thick

3 large parsnips, peeled and julienned, ½ cm (¼ inch) thick

2 tbsp maple syrup

Pinch of unrefined sea salt

Heat the oil in a pan over a medium heat. Add the julienned carrots and parsnips to the oil and stir continuously over a medium heat for about 5–6 minutes or until the vegetables become slightly tender. Note that some of the parsnips and carrots may become a little caramelized. Gently stir in the maple syrup and season with a pinch of salt. Continue to stir the carrots and parsnips for about 1–2 minutes or until the vegetables are well glazed by the maple syrup.

Caramelized Baked Pumpkin

1 large pumpkin, peeled, deseeded, center removed and cut into cubes

3 tbsp organic olive oil

Sea salt

2 tbsp maple sugar

Preheat oven to 220°C/425°F. Coat the pumpkin cubes with olive oil and sprinkle with sea salt and maple sugar. Cover with foil and bake for 15 minutes, then reduce the oven to 200°C/400°F and bake with the foil removed for a further 10 minutes, until the pumpkin caramelizes.

Turnip Delights

4 small turnips, washed, peeled and sliced in half

Sesame seeds

White miso

Lemon zest

Place the turnips in a large pan with just enough water to cover halfway. Bring to a boil and simmer for 15 minutes, until soft. Toast the sesame seeds until they pop, then grind them in a suribachi to form a paste (stopping before they turn to butter). Add two tablespoons of white miso, a small amount of water and the lemon zest, and mix together. When the turnips have cooled, scoop out a small part of the centers and stuff with the filling mixture.

Grain Dishes

Kasha Pilaf

1 cup uncooked kasha (buckwheat)

2 cups of Dashi Stock (see page 69)

2 tbsp olive oil

½ cup chopped onions

½ cup chopped mushrooms

2 tbsp minced fresh parsley

Roast the kasha in a pan until it is brown. Bring the dashi to a boil, add the kasha, turn down to a simmer and cook for 20 minutes. In a large pan, heat the olive oil and sauté the onions and mushrooms, adding a drop or two of shoyu. Add the sautéed vegetables to the kasha. Fluff with a fork and sprinkle with parsley. Serve with the Tahini-Béchamel Sauce on page 205.

Fried Rice Balls

Cooked short-grain
brown rice

Sunflower oil for frying

Shoyu

Form the rice into balls the size of a golf ball. Wet your hands in between to stop the rice from sticking to your fingers when rolling. Heat some oil in a heavy-based pan and fry the rice balls until slightly brown and crisp. Season with shoyu and eat hot.

Brown Rice with Millet or Barley

2 cups wholegrain brown rice, washed and soaked for minimum 1 hour

¼ cup barley or millet

4 cups water

2 pinches of sea salt

Place the rice with the barley or millet in a pressure cooker. When the water is warm, add the sea salt and put on the cover and bring to full pressure. Cook for about 45 minutes. Let sit for 5 minutes, then bring down the pressure and gently remove from the pot.

Shitake Wild Rice with Tahini-Béchamel Sauce

¾ cup brown rice, rinsed

¼ cup wild red rice, rinsed

1 chopped onion

3 cups chopped shitake mushrooms

1 tbsp toasted sesame oil

2–3 tsp tamari

1 cup chopped almonds

1 cup fresh parsley

Pinch of sea salt

Soak the grain in fresh spring water to cover for at least two and up to four hours, to help aid digestion of the grain.

Drain the water from the grain and place into the pressure cooker with one and a half cups of water. Bring to a boil with the lid loosely covered, then add the sea salt. Seal the lid and bring to full pressure. When the pressure comes up, immediately turn down to a low heat. Allow to cook for 30 minutes then turn off the heat and allow the pressure cooker to remain undisturbed for 25 minutes so that the rice continues to cook in its own heat. Remove the pot and transfer the rice to a serving bowl.

In a medium pan over a medium heat, sauté the onions and shitake mushrooms in sesame oil until the onions are soft and the mushrooms cooked. Add the tamari and simmer on a low heat for 5 minutes. Combine the mushrooms and onions with the rice and add the chopped almonds and parsley. Pour Tahini-Béchamel Sauce (see page 205) over the dish, mix and serve.

Tahini-Béchamel Sauce

2 tbsp tahini

4 tbsp water

4 tsp tamari

Pinch of sea salt

Mix the tahini and water in a small bowl. Add the tamari and salt, and mix.

Vegetable Barley Stew

Rice or barley stews seasoned with miso or umeboshi are the Japanese mother's cure-all. Maitake adds its healing and rejuvenating qualities to make this an even healthier dish.

1 cup barley, washed

½ cup dried maitake

12 cups water

1 piece kombu

1 tsp sea salt

1 bay leaf

½ tsp oregano

1 onion, diced

1 leek, sliced

2 large carrots, cut in half lengthwise, then into ½ cm (¼ inch) half moons

2 sticks celery, sliced

3 cups chopped kale or other leafy greens, such as chard or savoy cabbage

2–3 tbsp brown rice or barley miso

Chopped fresh parsley

Put the barley in a large saucepan with the maitake, water and kombu. Keep the mushrooms submerged by using a small plate or bowl on top, and soak for 1–3 hours. Take the kombu out and keep it for another time. Remove the maitake, chop finely and put back in the pan. Bring the liquid to the boil over a medium heat and add salt and a bay leaf. Lower the heat and simmer with the lid on but ajar, until the barley is tender. This will take about 45 minutes, plus an extra 20 minutes or so for a creamier texture.

Add oregano and all the vegetables except the greens. Simmer for 10 minutes. And the chopped greens and simmer for 15 minutes more. Remove from the heat. In a cup, dilute the miso in a little bit of hot water, then add it to the stew. Sprinkle with chopped parsley and serve.

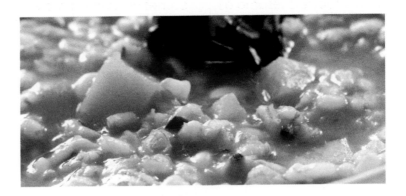

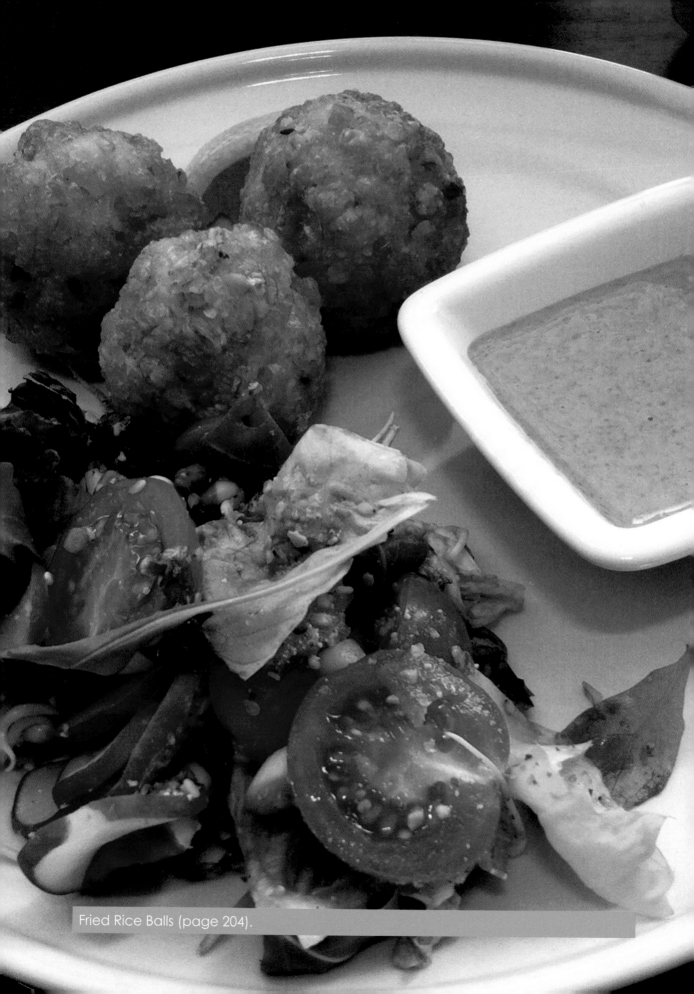

Fried Rice Balls (page 204).

Barley Cakes

2 garlic cloves, minced

2 leafy green leaves (e.g. collards, kale, bok choy), washed and thick stems removed

2 cups cooked pearled barley

1 medium onion, cut into small dice

½ cup fresh or frozen sweet peas

½ cup corn

1 cup cooked black soybeans, drained (or other beans)

½ cup daikon, washed and cut into ½ cm (¼ inch) dice

½ cup carrot, washed and cut into ½ cm (¼ inch) dice

¼ cup fresh parsley, washed and chopped

1 tbsp shoyu or tamari

1 cup organic white pastry flour

In a large sauté pan, toast the garlic in half a teaspoon of sesame oil. Remove the garlic from the oil and set aside. Stack the leafy greens and roll them like a cigar. Slice them very thinly. Heat some oil in the sauté pan over a medium-high flame and add the greens. Cook for 1 minute or until they are bright green. Remove the greens and set aside.

Place the cooked garlic, leafy greens, barley, onion, peas, corn, soybeans, daikon, carrot and parsley in a large bowl. Fold the mixture together until well blended. Add the tamari and flour. Test the mixture for ability to hold the shape of a small patty. If the mixture is too moist, add a small amount of flour and blend. If too dry, add water.

Brush the bottom of the sauté pan with sesame oil and heat over a medium flame. Place a food ring in the pan and spoon in the barley mixture. Pack the mixture in the ring, then remove the ring. Alternatively, shape the patty with the hands. Cook until golden brown on the bottom, turn over and cook until golden brown on both sides. For the garnish, drizzle with a dressing or sauce of your choice or create your own design. Sprinkle with fresh sliced scallions and toasted black sesame seeds.

Beans and Bean Products

Sweet and Sour Adzuki Beans

2 cups adzuki beans, soaked in cold water overnight with the kombu

15 cm (6 inch) piece kombu

¼ cup soy sauce

¼ cup olive or sesame oil

¼ cup apple cider vinegar

¼ cup rice syrup

2 onions, finely diced

Pressure cook the adzuki beans in the soaking water for 25 minutes. Alternatively bring the adzuki beans to a boil in the kombu soaking water. Cover and simmer for 45 minutes or until soft, adding more water if necessary. Preheat oven to 180°C/350°F. Mix the beans with the other ingredients in a bowl, blending well and then transfer to a baking dish. Cover the dish and bake in a medium-hot oven for 30 minutes. Remove the lid (if the beans look dry add some water) and bake for another 10–15 minutes. The onions and beans should be soft to the bite. Serve with cauliflower mash or polenta.

Fried Tofu

2 packets organic tofu, drained and cut into strips

3–4 tsp olive or sesame oil

2 bunches scallions

6 tsp rice flour

4 tsp freshly grated ginger juice

4 tsp shoyu

Pat the tofu slices dry with paper towels. Heat the oil in a heavy-bottomed frying pan and fry the scallions. Sprinkle the flour onto a plate. Place the tofu on the flour, coating the top and bottom of each strip. Fry until golden – about 3 minutes. Turn over and fry the other side. Add the ginger juice and shoyu to the pan and sizzle for a few more minutes. Serve with soba noodles or fried rice.

Tempeh with Tahini

2 onions, chopped

1 red bell pepper, deseeded and cut into small pieces

2 tsp oil

2 cups Dashi Stock (see page 69) or vegetable stock

2 tbsp miso mixed in a little water

200 g (7 oz) tempeh, cut in small cubes

1 tbsp umeboshi vinegar

1 tsp soy sauce

5 tbsp tahini

1 scallion, chopped

Sauté the onions and pepper in the oil in a pan. Add the dashi or vegetable stock, miso and tempeh and simmer for 40 minutes on a low heat, adding more liquid if necessary. Remove from the heat.

Mix the vinegar, soy sauce and tahini together, and add this to the pan. Garnish the tempeh with the chopped scallion. Serve hot with rice.

Alternatively you may purée the mixture with a hand blender to a creamy sauce and pour over hot noodles and top with steamed broccoli.

Sweet Red Beans

2 cups red beans of your choice

4 cups water

Piece of kombu (postage-stamp size)

Brown rice syrup

Pinch of sea salt

Place the beans in a pressure cooker with the water, add the salt and kombu, bring to full pressure then reduce the flame to low and cook for 45 minutes. When the pressure has come down, remove the lid and add the brown rice syrup to the beans. Serve with your choice of grains and vegetables. For quickness use canned organic beans.

Lentils with Squash

1 bay leaf

1 cup dried French green lentils

4 cups spring or filtered water

1 onion, diced

2 or 3 cups winter squash, cut into 1 cm (½ inch) cubes

Sea salt or soy sauce

Balsamic vinegar

Place the bay leaf, lentils and water in a pot, bring to a boil over a medium heat and boil uncovered for 10 minutes. Cover and cook over a low heat for 35 minutes, adding more water if required. Add the onion and squash and cook until the squash is tender – about 20 minutes or so. Season lightly with sea salt and simmer for 10 minutes. All the liquid should be absorbed and the stew should be creamy. Remove from the heat and sprinkle lightly with the balsamic vinegar. Mix well, transfer to a bowl and serve hot with your choice of cooked grain, such as wholegrain brown rice or millet, and sprinkle with sesame seeds. If you like, add a side dish of delicious greens, like broccoli or spinach, sautéed in olive oil or simply steamed or boiled. Alternatively, serve with a seaweed dish such as arame sauté.

Winter Bean and Kale Stew

¼ cup wakame

1 tbsp olive oil

1 small onion, diced

2 small carrots, diced

1 celery stalk, diced

1 can cannellini beans, rinsed and drained

1½ cups pinto beans (canned organic)

6 cups miso bouillon or 6 cups Dashi Stock (see page 69)

1 bunch kale, trimmed and chopped (6 cups)

¼ tsp dried oregano

⅛ to ¼ tsp ground nutmeg

Shoya or tamari to taste

Note: For a thicker stew-like consistency, add any choice of cooked grain to the pot such as millet, quinoa, barley, or short-grain rice.

Put the wakame in small bowl, cover with cold water and soak for 15 minutes, or until soft. Drain, squeeze out the liquid, cut into small pieces and set aside. Heat the oil in a saucepan over a medium heat. Add the onion, carrots, celery and wakame, and sauté for 3 to 5 minutes, or until tender. Add the cannellini beans, pinto beans and broth. Bring to a boil, reduce the heat to medium-low, cover and simmer for 10 minutes. Transfer half of the soup to a food processor or blender and purée until smooth. Stir the mixture into the remaining soup in the pot and add the kale. Cook for 5 minutes more, or until the kale is tender. Stir in the oregano and nutmeg and add a swirl or two of shoyu or tamari.

Sweet Black Bean Soup/Stew

1 cup black
soy beans

¼ cup sweet rice

2½ cups water

Piece of kombu
(postage-stamp size)

2 squares dried tofu

1 large carrot, cut into
shaved chunks

1 onion, cut into cubes

Barley miso

Sunflower oil

Scallions

Soak the tofu in water. Roast the beans in a pressure cooker until the skins begin to crack open. Add the kombu and one-third or one-quarter of a cup of sweet rice. Add twice the amount of water. Bring to pressure and cook for 50 minutes. Squeeze the water from the tofu. Cut the tofu into cubes and deep fry in sunflower oil for 30 seconds to 1 minute.

When the beans and rice are cooked and the pressure is down, remove the kombu, add the tofu, carrots and onions and more water, and bring to a boil. Simmer for approximately 10 to 15 minutes until the vegetables are tender. Just before the vegetables are cooked, add the miso (dilute first in a little water). Simmer very gently for 4 minutes. Serve in a bowl with scallion to garnish.

Tempeh Kebabs with Peanut Sauce

You can replace the tempeh with tofu for a different taste and texture.

1 pack tempeh, cut into
equal squares

1 zucchini, sliced

1 carrot, sliced

1 onion, cubed, or baby
onions

1 red pepper, cubed

Mushrooms, brushed and
cleaned

Preheat oven to 190°C/375°F. Using skewers, make the kebabs with one or two pieces of each of the above ingredients. Place the kebabs on a baking tray with parchment paper and drizzle olive oil over them. Cook for around 25 minutes, turning them over halfway through the cooking time. Remove and drizzle balsamic vinegar over the kebabs and continue to cook for a further 10 minutes. Serve on a bed of grains of your choice, such as quinoa, bulgur or couscous, and drizzle Peanut Sauce (see page 213) over the top. Serve with a crisp, fresh green salad.

Breakfast or Sandwich Tempeh

½ cup water

2 tbsp miso paste

2 cloves garlic, thinly sliced

1 tbsp mustard

2 bay leaves

¼ tsp white pepper

1 pack tempeh, cut into thin strips

Sesame oil

Boil the water in a medium saucepan and stir in the miso until it is diluted. Add the garlic, mustard, bay leaves and pepper. Add the tempeh strips, cover the pan and simmer for 20 minutes. Preheat the grill. Remove the tempeh strips and place them on a lightly oiled baking sheet. Grill the strips for 5 to 8 minutes until they are crisp and golden brown on one side. Turn the strips over and cook for another 5 minutes, before serving on wholegrain bread spread with vegan mayonnaise. Top with some salad greens and sauerkraut.

Sauces, Salads and Side Dishes

Double Cranberry Chutney

2 tbsp fresh orange juice

1 tbsp fresh lemon juice

1 tsp arrowroot powder

½ tsp dry mustard

4 cups fresh or frozen cranberries

1½ cups rice syrup

½ cup dried cranberries

3 tbsp finely crystallized ginger

2 tbsp grated orange zest

1 tbsp grated lemon zest

⅛ tsp ground cloves

Pinch of sea salt

Whisk together the orange juice, lemon juice, arrowroot and mustard in a small bowl, then set aside. Combine the cranberries, rice syrup, dried cranberries, ginger, orange zest, lemon zest, cloves and a pinch of sea salt in a medium saucepan. Bring to a boil, while stirring. Stir in the arrowroot mixture, reduce the heat to medium-low and simmer for 10 to 15 minutes, or until the sauce thickens and the berries have burst. Cool and serve chilled or at room temperature. Serve with Grain Burgers (see page 75).

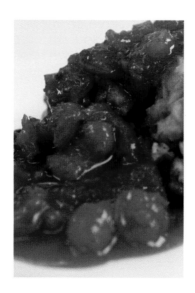

Carrot and Tahini Spread

2 large carrots, cut into small pieces

½ cup water

1–2 tbsp tahini

Pinch of sea salt

Put the carrots in a saucepan and add salt and water. Simmer on a medium flame until the carrots are soft enough to be mashed. When ready, remove the carrots from the pot and purée them with a hand blender or mash by hand, to reach a creamy consistency using some of the water in which they were cooked. Add the tahini and mix well. Sprinkle with toasted sesame seeds. Serve on crepes, toast or rice cakes, or over grains.

Peanut Sauce

2 tsp avocado or other vegetable oil

1 tbsp grated onion

1 clove fresh garlic, finely minced

2 tsp chilli powder (if hot/spicy taste desired)

1 cup unsweetened organic peanut butter

1 tbsp brown rice syrup

Juice of 1 lemon

Soy sauce

Spring or filtered water

Heat the oil in a small pan. Add the onion, garlic and chilli powder (if using), and cook, while stirring, over a medium heat for 2 to 3 minutes. Add the peanut butter, a dash of soy sauce and the rice syrup. Stir well and simmer over a very low heat for 5 minutes. Remove from the heat and stir in the lemon juice and enough water to obtain the desired consistency of the sauce.

The dips below make tasty festive season snacks. Oven-crisped and lightly seasoned roasted root vegetables make for a healthy appetizer option that won't overpower the other foods served.

Garlic-Bean Dip

Roasting the garlic helps mellow its flavor in this dip.

6 medium carrots, trimmed, peeled and cut into sticks (6 cups)

6 medium beetroots, peeled and cut into carrot-like sticks (6 cups)

2½ tbsp olive oil, divided

1 head garlic

1 can cannellini beans, drained and liquid reserved

1 tbsp lemon juice

1 tsp grated lemon zest

1 tsp dried basil

Preheat oven to 230°C/450°F. Toss the carrots and beetroots with one and a half tablespoons of oil and season with salt and pepper, if desired. Spread the vegetables in a single layer on a baking sheet. Trim the papery top from the head of the garlic, just to the cloves. Wrap it in foil and place in the corner of the baking sheet. Roast the vegetables and garlic for 25 minutes, or until the carrots and beetroots are tender, but not soft, and the garlic packet feels soft when lightly squeezed. Remove the baking sheet from the oven, open the foil packet around the garlic, and allow the vegetables and garlic to cool.

Squeeze the garlic cloves from their skins and place in a food processor with the cannellini beans, lemon juice, lemon zest, basil and remaining one tablespoon of oil. Pulse the mixture until creamy and smooth, adding some reserved bean liquid, if necessary. Season with salt and pepper, if desired. Serve in a bowl alongside roasted vegetables.

Avocado Cream Dip

2 ripe avocados, peeled and sliced

Juice of 1 lemon

1 tsp salt

1 tsp umeboshi paste

2 tbsp olive oil

Put all the ingredients in a bowl and mix with a hand blender to a creamy texture. Adjust seasoning to taste. Serve with oatcakes or crudités.

White Bean Dip

2 tbsp plus 1 tsp olive oil

1 medium onion, chopped

1 tbsp minced garlic

½ tsp salt

½ tsp freshly ground black pepper

2 tsp finely chopped fresh rosemary

2 cans cannellini beans, rinsed and drained

1 tbsp white wine vinegar

1 tbsp dry breadcrumbs, plus extra breadcrumbs for topping

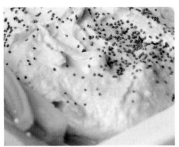

Preheat oven to 180°C/350°F. Heat one tablespoon of oil in a medium saucepan over a medium heat. Add the onion and garlic and cook for about 8 minutes, until translucent. Add the salt and pepper and one teaspoon of rosemary – stir well to combine. Scrape into a food processor fitted with the steel blade. Transfer the beans to the food processor bowl and add the vinegar, one tablespoon of olive oil and three tablespoons of water. Purée until smooth. Combine the breadcrumbs, remaining rosemary and remaining olive oil in a small bowl, and stir until combined. Place the bean purée in an ovenproof bowl and top with the breadcrumb mixture. Transfer to the oven and bake until golden brown – about 20 minutes. Serve with roasted vegetables.

Mock Tuna

Tuna is very yang and contracting – considered too strong an energy to take in regularly, especially for a woman. This is also true for salmon. Macrobiotic recipes generally stick to white-fleshed fish, which are lower in fat and more easily digestible. Therefore, to imitate the sensual pleasure of tuna fish, we use tempeh.

1 pack tempeh

1 tbsp umeboshi vinegar

⅓ cup Tofu Mayonnaise (see page 217)

1 celery stalk, diced

¼ red onion, finely diced

Any spices you desire such as cumin, paprika, saffron, etc. (optional)

Black pepper to taste (if desired)

Steam or boil the tempeh for 20 minutes to make it more digestible. Break it apart with a fork until you get smaller than bite-sized pieces. Sprinkle the umeboshi vinegar onto the tempeh, mashing it in with a fork until you get a tuna-fishy saltiness. Mix the Tofu Mayonnaise, pepper and any other spices you enjoy. Mash into the tempeh, then add the celery and onion. Serve or refrigerate – it tastes even better the next day.

Chickpea and Artichoke Wraps

6 barley tortillas (e.g. Mountain Bread) or rice tortillas

Filling

1¼ cups green cabbage, very thinly sliced

2 medium carrots, shredded (¾ cup)

½ medium green bell pepper, very thinly sliced

3 tbsp Tofu Mayonnaise (see page 217)

1 tbsp chopped fresh parsley

1 tbsp minced red onion

2 tsp fresh lemon juice

¼ tsp salt

¼ tsp freshly ground pepper

Artichoke Spread

1 can artichoke hearts, drained and halved

1 cup canned chickpeas, rinsed and drained

⅓ cup tahini

Small handful fresh parsley leaves

1 medium clove garlic, coarsely chopped

1 tbsp fresh lemon juice

½ tsp salt

⅛ to ¼ tsp freshly ground pepper

Combine all the ingredients for the Artichoke Spread and two tablespoons of water in a food processor or blender. Process until the mixture is almost smooth, but retains some texture and is slightly thicker than hummus. If necessary, add more water with a teaspoon to thin. Adjust the seasonings to taste.

For the filling, in a medium bowl combine the cabbage, carrots, bell pepper, Tofu Mayonnaise, parsley, onion, lemon juice, salt and pepper. Mix well. In a large pan, warm each tortilla over a medium heat just until soft and flexible – about 1 minute per side. Spread some of the artichoke mixture over each tortilla, leaving a finger-width border. Top with the cabbage mixture, dividing equally. Fold the bottom end of the tortilla partially over the filling, then roll into a bundle and serve.

Tofu Mayonnaise

1 packet of soft or silken tofu, sliced into 4 pieces

3 tbsp apple cider vinegar

1 tbsp rice syrup

4 tbsp olive oil

½ tsp sea salt

2 tsp Dijon mustard

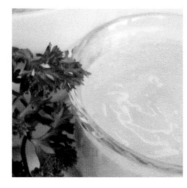

Steam the tofu for 5 minutes and allow it to cool. In a small pot, gently warm the cider vinegar, rice syrup, oil, salt and mustard over a medium-high heat for 2 to 3 minutes, being careful not to let the liquid boil. Transfer to a blender and blend all the ingredients until creamy.

Pumpkin Cream

A more unusual way to eat pumpkin – but delicious nonetheless. A tasty treat during the Christmas holidays.

1 large pumpkin, peeled, seeded and cubed

1 cup maple sugar

1 tbsp organic olive oil

Zest of ½ orange

Juice and zest of 1 lemon

Place the pumpkin in a pan and add water to cover the base. Stew until the pumpkin is soft, adding more water if necessary and stirring regularly to ensure it doesn't stick. Once the pumpkin has collapsed, add the sugar, olive oil, orange zest, lemon zest and juice. Cook rapidly until the mixture thickens. Pot in jars and enjoy over the festive season.

See photograph on page 218.

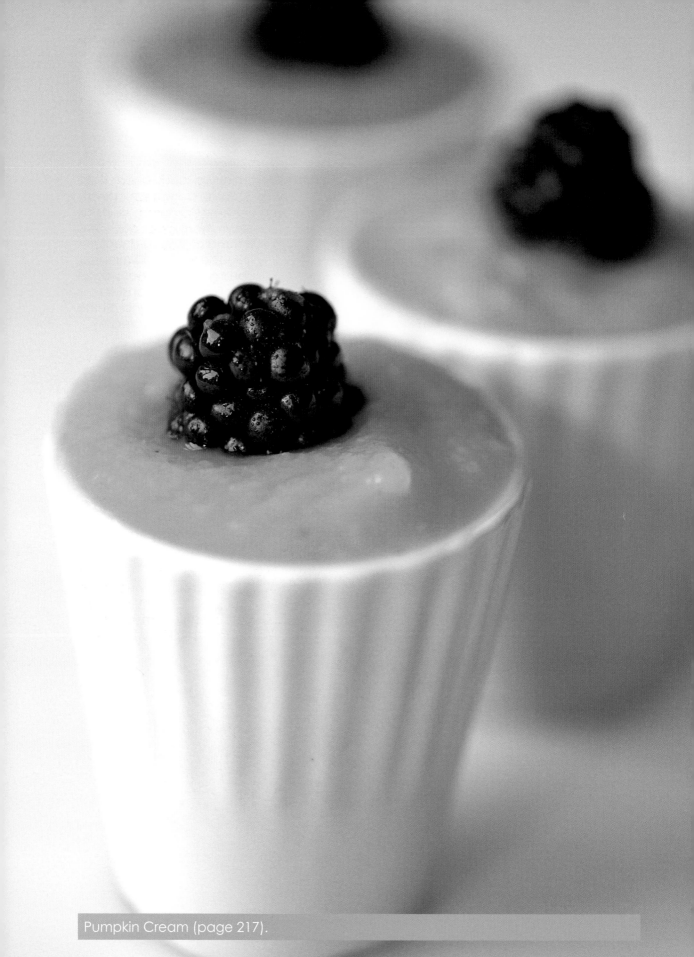

Pumpkin Cream (page 217).

Zucchini and Avocado Hummus

1 tbsp warm water and lemon juice from ½ lemon

¼ cup tahini

½ avocado, peeled, cored and mashed

½ cup carrots, shredded

2 zucchini, shredded

1 can organic garbanzo beans, drained and rinsed

¼ cup sweet onion, chopped

1 tbsp rice syrup

¼ tsp chilli powder (optional)

In a food processor, combine the lemon juice, water and tahini, and purée until a smooth consistency is reached. Slowly add the mashed avocado, shredded carrots, and shredded zucchini, and continue to purée. Add the garbanzo beans, chopped onion, rice syrup and chilli powder (if using). Purée until it forms the desired smooth consistency. Transfer into serving dishes. Enjoy with your favorite wholegrain chips, pita bread, crackers or raw vegetables.

Popcorn

½ cup popcorn kernels

3 tbsp sesame oil

Refined sea salt

Heat the oil in a heavy-bottomed pan and add the popcorn kernels. Put the lid on and turn the heat right up. Once the oil begins to heat up, the corn will start popping. When the popping stops, the corn is ready. Serve the popcorn in a bowl and sprinkle with some refined sea salt.

Nori Condiment

5–6 sheets toasted nori, cut into 2½ cm (1 inch) pieces

½ cup water

½ small onion, finely chopped

1 clove garlic, crushed

2 tbsp tamari

Juice squeezed from 1 small piece ginger

Few drops toasted sesame oil

Cover the nori with half a cup of water in a small saucepan. Soak for 10 minutes. Heat the saucepan and add the onion, garlic and two tablespoons of tamari. Bring to a boil and simmer for 30 minutes, stirring often until the water has evaporated and the nori forms a thick paste. Grate a small piece of ginger and squeeze the juice and a few drops of toasted sesame oil into the pan. Lower the heat right down and continue cooking and stirring for a few more minutes. Cool and store in a glass jar in the refrigerator for up to 5 days.

Pressed Salad

Assortment of fresh vegetables

Sea salt

Wash and slice the vegetables into very thin slices. I use a mandolin for quickness. In a large bowl, mix the vegetables and add about half a teaspoon of sea salt per cup of chopped vegetables. Mix gently by hand. Transfer to a salad press and apply pressure to the press. Let the vegetables sit for one hour or more (depending on the vegetables), or until water is expelled from the vegetables. Discard the water before serving and rinse off the vegetables under fresh water if they taste too salty. Serve plain or with lemon juice, rice vinegar or umeboshi vinegar.

For tasty salads try the following, pressed for 30 minutes:

✿ mustard greens or radish greens – chopped finely

✿ cabbage leaves – finely chopped and layered with sea salt

✿ carrots – grated, shredded or cut into matchsticks

Ingredients may be pressed longer – up to a couple of days – to make light pickles. Brown rice vinegar, umeboshi vinegar or shoyu may be used instead of salt, for variety in the pressing.

Desserts

Chocolate Pudding

3 tbsp arrowroot powder or kuzu

2 tbsp water

1½ cups almond milk

Seeds from 1 vanilla pod

¼ cup brown rice syrup

¼ cup unsweetened cocoa powder

Pinch of sea salt

Form a paste by combining the arrowroot or kuzu and water in a cup. Whisk all the ingredients, including the arrowroot mixture, in a small saucepan and bring to a slow boil. Using the whisk, continue stirring until the mixture comes to a boil and starts to thicken. Remove from the heat and allow to set for a few hours in a flat dish. Place the mixture in a blender and purée to a smooth cream. Pour into small glass serving cups and top with some crushed nuts and non-dairy whipped cream.

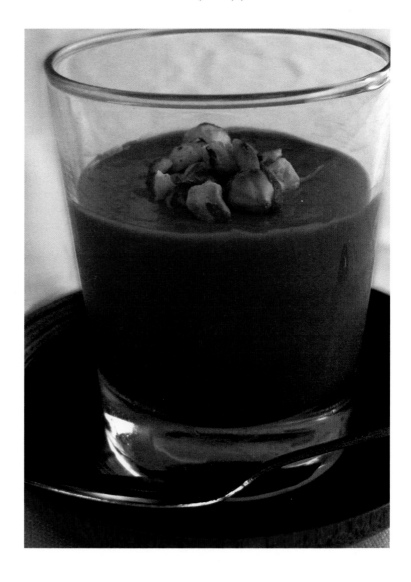

Rice Pudding

1 cup amasake (or rice milk)

½ cup apple juice

2 cups cooked brown rice

3 tbsp raisins

3 tbsp sunflower seeds

1 tsp cinnamon

1 tsp vanilla

Combine all the ingredients except the vanilla in a large saucepan. Simmer over a medium-low heat for 20 to 30 minutes, stirring often to prevent sticking, until thick and creamy. Stir in the vanilla and serve warm or chilled.

Coconut Macaroons with Chocolate Glaze

Macaroons

2½ cups unsweetened, shredded coconut

⅓ cup wholewheat pastry flour

½ tsp baking powder

⅓ cup brown rice syrup

½ tsp pure almond extract

⅔ cup almond milk

Pinch of sea salt

Chocolate Glaze

½ cup grain-sweetened non-dairy chocolate chips

2–3 tbsp almond milk

2 tsp brown rice syrup

Preheat oven to 200°C/400°F. Line two baking sheets with parchment paper. Combine all the ingredients for the coconut macaroons, mixing well. Set aside so the coconut can absorb the liquid – about 5 minutes. You should have a thick batter, but it will not be very cohesive. Drop the batter by teaspoonfuls onto the baking sheets, and form into peaked cookies with your fingers. Bake for about 20 minutes, or until the coconut begins to brown. Transfer to a wire rack to cool.

For the glaze, place the chocolate chips in a heat-resistant bowl. Combine the almond milk and rice syrup in a small saucepan and bring to a full boil. Pour over the chocolate and whisk until smooth and satiny. Transfer to a plastic squeeze bottle. Slip a piece of parchment paper under the wire rack. Moving in a zigzag direction, drizzle the cookies with the glaze. Leave to stand for a few minutes to allow the glaze to set.

Orange and Walnut Adzuki Truffles

1 cup cooked adzuki beans

1 heaped tbsp hazelnut butter

2 tbsp rice syrup

½ tsp vanilla essence

Zest of 1 orange

Ground walnuts

Grain-based chocolate chips

Blend the adzuki beans, hazelnut butter, rice syrup and vanilla either by hand or using a hand blender. Place the mixture in a bowl and add enough ground walnuts to form dough that sticks and binds together. Stir in the orange zest. Roll into small truffle-sized balls.

Add a coating of your choice – melted grain-based chocolate chips, desiccated coconut, cocoa powder, sesame seeds or finely chopped dried fruit and nut mixture. Chill in the refrigerator. To melt the grain-based chocolate chips, simply place in a heat-proof bowl atop a pan of simmering water to attain a smooth liquid.

Fat-Free Brownies

Applesauce is used in place of oil.

Brownies

1½ cups wholewheat pastry flour

3 tbsp cocoa

1½ tsp baking powder

1 tsp baking soda

¼ tsp sea salt

½ cup sugar free chocolate chips

½ cup brown rice syrup

2 tsp vanilla

½ cup apple sauce

1 cup water

Topping

¼ cup vanilla rice milk

1 tsp vanilla

½ cup applesauce

½ cup brown rice syrup

½ cup cocoa

Preheat oven to 200°C/400°F. Oil a 23×28 cm (9×11–inch) Pyrex dish. For the brownies, sift the dry ingredients. Mix the wet ingredients and add together, mixing well. Bake for 15 minutes then reduce the heat to 150°C/300°F and bake for another 5 minutes. Remove and allow to cool. Cut into small squares.

For the topping, combine the ingredients and simmer while stirring. Pour over the cooled brownies and serve with some Tofu and Vanilla Whip (see page 153).

Orange-Ginger Oatmeal Crunch Cookies

1½ cups oatmeal

¾ cup wholewheat pastry flour

¾ cup unbleached white flour

1 tsp baking powder

½ tsp sea salt

¾ cup currants

1 cup walnuts, toasted and coarsely chopped

½ cup walnut oil

½ cup barley malt or brown rice syrup

Zest of 1 orange

½ cup orange juice

1 tbsp peeled and finely grated fresh ginger

1 tsp vanilla

Preheat oven to 180°C/350°F. Line two baking sheets with parchment or brush with oil. In a medium-large bowl, mix the dry ingredients. In a smaller bowl, whisk together the wet ingredients then stir into the dry ingredients. Makes 3 cups batter.

Transfer heaping tablespoons of dough to a baking sheet, leaving at least an inch of space between the cookies. If uniformity is important, use a one-quarter or one-third cup scoop. Flatten the cookies with the back of a fork to make round shapes, eight to ten centimeters (three to four inches) in diameter and one centimeter (half an inch) thick. Dip the scoop and/or fork in water to keep the mixture from sticking. Bake the cookies until the edges and undersides are golden – 25 to 30 minutes.

Festive Granola Bars

2½ cups rolled oats

1 cup wholewheat pastry flour

½ tsp baking soda

½ tsp salt, divided

⅔ cup chopped dried apricots

½ cup unsweetened chocolate chips

½ cup chopped walnuts

1 cup packed maple sugar

½ cup maple syrup

½ cup almond butter

¼ cup vegetable oil

½ cup tofu, mashed

Preheat oven to 180°C/350°F. Coat a 23×33 cm (9×13–inch) baking dish with a small drop of oil. Combine the oats, flour, baking soda and one-quarter teaspoon of salt in a bowl. Stir in the apricots, chocolate chips and walnuts. Beat the maple sugar, maple syrup, almond butter, oil and tofu until smooth. Stir in the oat mixture.

Spread the mixture in a prepared baking dish and pat down firmly. Sprinkle the top with the remaining salt. Bake for 30 to 35 minutes, or until firm. Cool for 20 minutes before slicing into bars.

Seaweed Nut Crunch

¼ cup sesame oil

½ cup maple syrup

1 cup sliced almonds

1 cup sesame seeds

6 sheets of nori seaweed, torn into little pieces

1 tsp shoyu

Preheat oven to 180°C/350°F. Pour the oil and maple syrup into a large pan. Bring to a frothy boil and add the sliced almonds, stir, and add the sesame seeds and nori pieces. Sprinkle in the shoyu. Continue stirring until everything is coated. Pour into one layer on a baking sheet and bake for 10 minutes. Allow to cool and cut into slices.

Pears with Ginger Glaze and Pecan Cream

Pecan Cream

2 cups pecans

1 cup soy milk

¼ cup rice syrup

2 tsp vanilla extract

½ tsp umeboshi vinegar

Pears

4 pears, peeled, cored and halved

2 cups organic pear juice (set aside ¼ cup for diluting the kuzu)

1 tsp ginger juice

1 tbsp kuzu (dissolved in a little water)

8 sprigs fresh mint for garnish

Preheat oven to 180°C/350°F. For the Pecan Cream, place the pecans on a baking tray and bake 10 minutes. Transfer the toasted pecans to a food processor and grind into a powder. Add the remaining ingredients to the food processor and blend till smooth. Refrigerate for 30 minutes.

Place the pears in a pan. Add the pear juice and ginger juice, bring to a boil, then cover, reduce heat and simmer for about 10 minutes, or until the pears are soft. Remove the pears and place in individual serving dishes. Thicken the leftover juice in the bottom of the pan with the diluted kuzu, stirring constantly to avoid lumping. Add pear juice as required for the desired consistency. Pour the kuzu glaze over the pears, add a spoonful or two of Pecan Cream, and garnish with a sprig of fresh mint.

Chapter 11

MAKING CHANGE – QUICK AND EASY

Relax and Take a Deep Breath – I Have the Answers You Need!

I suggest to all of my clients and students that they begin by setting themselves a goal that they feel is possible to reach, and then move towards it. For example, in (say) 3 months' time I will have a kitchen free of sugar, dairy and animal food (or whatever it is you want to eliminate). Write down the steps you need to take to get you there.

Check out the local supermarket and natural food store for healthy alternatives. Start reading labels. Many of the foods labelled "healthy" contain fructose and other forms of processed chemicals and additives, so anything with more than three or four syllables in it is made by a chemist and not by Mother Nature. I have created a shopping-list guide below to help you.

Connect with people who are also eating a healthy diet. It is not always possible to make an immediate change, especially when families are involved, who might have differing views. You can slowly move towards your goal by introducing new foods, rather than immediately throwing away the processed and sugared ones that your family members are eating. Some clients prefer to start full on, while others prefer to take it more slowly – decide what suits you.

When shopping, buy organic produce and sugar-free jams, biscuits and juices. Gradually replace the processed items with those of better quality, such as sea salt, brown rice vinegar, sesame and olive oils, and sourdough wholewheat bread or sprouted bread.

When it comes to cooking the meals, begin to include more vegetables and whole grains. Try a new recipe that might appeal to your family, such as fried noodles or fried rice, once or twice a week. Incorporate the quick basic recipes given later in this chapter, to get you started.

Soups are always a popular choice. You can add miso to almost any bean or vegetable soup. You will be surprised how a small shift in direction will produce great results. If members of your family are willing to try the new foods, they will also begin to change their diet naturally, without it being forced upon them.

Change often seems more difficult than it actually is, and the constant thinking about it is what causes us to get stuck. Once you create action by starting to put things into practice, life becomes much easier. There is no correct way to change your diet and lifestyle – it is whatever suits you and your family. Suggest to your family that they also become involved in this new way of eating, and research the effect of food on their health. It is widely recognized that we need to make more effort to provide a healthy diet for our families and ourselves.

Dishes such as adzuki bean stew with kombu seaweed, or maitake or shitake teas that I make for clients, are incredible for regulating the function of the kidneys, softening them so they can do their job (which is to detox) efficiently. The teas also aid in weight loss, working deep within the body to restore balance: they help to dissolve the fat while adding minerals to increase blood quality. Kombu seaweed, for example, helps to balance the functioning of the nervous system, which of course includes the brain. There is tremendous power in these incredible foods.

Utensils

The one thing we use in macrobiotic cooking is a pressure cooker for cooking whole grains, beans and stew dishes. A Japanese vegetable knife for cutting is necessary, and a suribachi (Japanese grinding bowl) is indispensable for making gomashio (natural sea salt condiment). A salad press is a useful utensil for making quick pickles. Glass jars are a perfect way of storing all your grains and beans, as well as making a wonderful display in your kitchen.

How Do We Create Incredible Energy in Our Food?

1 Pick the highest quality, locally grown, seasonally available, freshest ingredients.

2 Choose organically grown food.

3 Cook whole grains or beans under pressure, i.e. in a pressure cooker.

4 Use stainless steel and natural cookware (no aluminium pots or pans).

5 Cook preferably with gas rather than electricity – no microwaving.

6 Use a slightly higher flame.

7 Use a slightly longer time for cooking or aging.

8 Use only sea salt or natural seasonings such as tamari or shoyu.

9 Cook dynamically with a variety of foods, styles, colors, tastes and textures – creamy, crunchy, chewy and other energies.

10 Cook with love and a calm, peaceful mind.

11 Thoroughly chew each mouthful of food.

12 Eat with gratitude.

The way of eating is just as important as the food itself. Keeping meals peaceful and relaxed and eating at regular times is especially relevant.

List of Ingredients for a Healthy Transition to a Natural Wholefood Diet

Instead of …	Use …
Baked goods	Sugar and dairy-free cookies and muffins
Black teas	Bancha twig tea (kukicha) or other medicinal teas
White bread	Wholegrain, sourdough or sprouted bread
Cheese products	Mochi (sweet brown rice) or finely grated roasted tofu
Meat	Seitan (wheat meat), textured vegetable protein (TVP), tempeh or tofu
Meat stock	Miso, miso bouillon, dulse or vegetable stock
Milk	Rice, oat or almond milk
Pasta dishes	Wholewheat, rice or spelt pasta, or soba noodles
Iodized salt	Natural sea salt
White rice	Short-grain brown rice or other whole grain
Sugar	Brown rice syrup or barley malt syrup
Scrambled eggs	Tofu (scrambles well)
Soy sauce (commercial)	Shoyu or tamari (naturally fermented soy sauce)

Quick Bites and Leftovers

Cook Once – Eat Twice

Time-savers are a great way to cook your food. Cook double the quantity and use half for tomorrow's lunch. Prepare more than you need and freeze the rest. A good idea is to freeze in small portions so that you have "ready-made" meals when you are pressed for time.

✿ Make double the amount of a sauce and use for another dish later in the week.

✿ Freeze half to use for future quick dinners.

✿ Use up any leftover vegetables to make a juice.

✿ Wash and cut up enough fresh vegetables for meals for several days. Keep the cut vegetables in sealed containers in the fridge, so that most of the preparation is done and you can cook a meal quickly. This is not ideal, but it's better than eating take-out.

✿ Alternatively, peel and chop carrots, onions, or other veggies, bag them and freeze. When needed, just take out as much as you require and reseal. No more soggy vegetables at the bottom of your vegetable box.

✿ Organize a weekly menu plan – this makes it possible to efficiently use leftovers and simplifies meal preparation.

✿ Beans and grains will last for three days after being cooked. Cook enough beans to use in a stew or casserole and also for adding to a minestrone soup. Brown rice (or any grain) can accompany vegetables with a nut or seed garnish; it can be fried with vegetables in a stir-fry or made into porridge by adding water. Grains and beans are fine to reuse but the vegetables must be fresh.

✿ Make a large soup stock with vegetables and wakame seaweed and keep it in the fridge. Purée a little miso with water and set aside. When you want soup, simply use the required quantity of stock and heat well. Then put some of the miso in the bottom of the bowl and pour the stock over it, stir and serve.

✿ Sea vegetable dishes keep well for several days. Cook up a good batch and then use a small portion daily.

✿ Always have some wholegrain pasta (spelt is good), bulgur, couscous and other partially refined grains at hand for last-minute meals.

✿ Learn how to make a few delicious vegetarian sauces and dressings. Make some up and keep them in the fridge. That way you can always put together quick salads or other dishes and dress them up.

✿ Have a stock of organic cooked beans and other foods at hand for when you get stuck.

✿ Choose two new recipes from your cookbooks every week so that you are constantly expanding your range of dishes and your familiarity with the foods.

The kitchen cupboard is the nerve center of your kitchen – keep it well stocked and you will save time, avoiding a dash to the shops for that single missing ingredient; you will always have a delicious meal at hand, even when the fridge is looking bare. Canned organic beans are a great addition to soups and make tasty dips.

Shortcuts to Healthy Eating for Busy People

Most people think you are tied to the kitchen when you eat the macrobiotic way, but if you organize yourself well you can spend literally 20 minutes in the kitchen and have a delicious meal ready, by having prepped and stored various items like vegetables, grains, bean dishes and soups beforehand. As you will see from the above quick bites, a breakfast, lunch or dinner can be put together in no time at all. It is all about planning ahead and being organized. Storing and reheating cooked food makes it possible to serve delicious healthy meals in as little as 10 minutes. "Cook once, eat twice" is my motto. Using soba, udon, quick-cooking grains, or lightly boiled or steamed vegetables are all easy ways to cook up something tasty in no time.

Breakfast

Here are some quick breakfast tips. Heat some leftover whole grains into porridge and add seeds, nuts and dried or stewed fruit of your choice. Or toast or steam some sourdough bread and spread some almond paste, peanut spread or tahini on it – delicious! Slice an apple and have a serving of some toasted pumpkin or sunflower seeds with it. Make a green juice or other fresh fruit or vegetable juice. Bancha twig tea can be made in batches so you only need to add some boiling water to it. At the weekends, when time is not of the essence, cook some scrambled tofu and serve with a toasted baguette, or make some wholewheat pancakes with blueberries. Personally I always start the day with a bowl of miso soup to alkalize my blood and then have some porridge.

Lunch

Heat up some leftover soup. Make enough soup for 3 or 4 days and take some from the fridge when you need it. Steam or fry leftover grains or make sushi with the rice. Refer to the leftover rice ideas on page 234; these can also be used for rice that has been prepared earlier. Keep some rice balls stored in the fridge for a snack attack. Any grain, such as quinoa, served with a fresh green salad and some tofu dressing can be a delightful lunch. Sauerkraut and cucumber sandwiches topped with tempeh on sourdough bread are quick and tasty, as are bean pâtés with some fresh greens. Falafel is a good choice for lunch, alongside a fresh green salad. The list of delicious lunches you can put together using leftovers is quite incredible.

Dinner

Use leftover bean stew or nishime by reheating and serving with some freshly cooked vegetables and a grain or noodle of your choice. A tempeh and seitan pan-fry is ready in a few minutes and can be served with a sauce or dressing made previously and stored in the refrigerator. Sautéed baby bok choy with fresh shitake mushrooms takes only minutes to cook – serve with leftover whole grains and top with almonds, again using one of the leftover sauces/dressings. This makes a tasty meal with the minimum of effort. Refer to your recipes and start creating your own dishes.

Try one or two of the following to add freshness to your leftovers:

✿   Pressed salad

✿   Sauerkraut

❀   Watercress and dulse salad

❀   Blanched vegetables

❀   Steamed vegetables

Once you become familiar with all the ingredients, you can whip up a delicious, healthy lunch or dinner for family and friends like a professional chef, with the minimum of effort. There are many readily available ingredients that will also enable you to make a healthy macrobiotic meal quickly, such as mochi, tofu, natto, tempeh, seitan, natural pesto sauces, sauerkraut, hummus, and vegetable, bean or grain burgers.

Quick Dishes That Take Only 10 Minutes

Quick Rice

1–2 tsp olive or sesame oil

5 cm (2 inch) piece of ginger, very finely chopped

2 or 3 cloves garlic, very finely chopped

200 g (2 cups) cooked short-grain brown rice

Sea salt

Parsley, finely chopped

Heat the oil in a wok and add the ginger and garlic, stirring constantly. Add the cooked rice and stir quickly over a high heat for a few minutes, then add the salt and stir for another couple of minutes. Mix thoroughly and transfer to a serving dish. Garnish with parsley and serve.

Quick Miso Soup

4 cups filtered water

5 cm (2 inch) piece dried wakame

1 onion, thinly sliced

Handful of watercress, finely chopped

2 bok choy leaves, finely chopped

Scallions, finely chopped

Barley miso

Soak the wakame for 5 minutes and cut into small pieces. Add the wakame to filtered water and bring to a boil. Add the onion and simmer for 5 minutes. Reduce the flame to low. Dilute the miso in a little water (1 teaspoon per cup of broth), add to the soup and simmer on a low heat for 3 to 4 minutes. Add the watercress and bok choy leaves and turn off the heat. If you desire, serve with strips of nori or add a pinch of grated ginger. Top with the scallion.

Great Ideas for Using Leftover Brown Rice

✿ Steam the rice in a steamer with diced carrots, corn and peas. Sprinkle with toasted walnuts for garnish. Use other vegetables and nuts for variety.

✿ Steam the rice and then layer it with re-fried beans – it takes only 10 minutes. Serve with some fresh greens.

✿ Rice balls with a dab of tahini or umeboshi and wrapped in a strip of nori is a daily staple of mine. Roll the rice in your hand to form a ball the size of a golf ball. Make a hole in the middle with your thumb and put some umeboshi paste, tahini or peanut butter inside. Roll in toasted sesame seeds or wrap in a sheet of nori cut into half. Wet your fingers and roll the nori around the rice ball to seal.

✿ Pan-fried rice with sesame oil, shoyu and ginger is a quick and satisfying meal. You can also add some tofu, tempeh or seitan.

✿ Pan-fried rice with olive oil, garlic and broccoli, served with one of the delicious dressings, is a tasty and fulfilling side dish, or add a can of organic chickpeas to make a complete meal.

✿ Miso soup becomes a meal when you add leftover cooked short-grain rice, millet or quinoa. I often use soba or udon noodles, which then turn a simple bowl of miso into a very satisfying meal. Serve with a fresh green salad on the side.

✿ Soft rice porridge with a sweet or savory taste is a great way to start the day.

✿ Try sushi using different fillings, such as peanut butter and sauerkraut, tahini with umeboshi, or cucumber with avocado and shiso – the possibilities are endless. Be creative and have fun experimenting with the tastes and textures. Creamy, crunchy and chewy is what we need for satisfaction.

✿ Brown rice pudding with tahini, rice syrup, apple juice, chopped almonds and raisins is nature's perfect comfort food. Use leftover rice, warm in a small pan with some apple juice, and add a small amount of tahini or rice syrup. Sprinkle with the almonds and raisins.

A–Z OF MACROBIOTIC SUPERFOODS

Some of the listed natural ingredients may already be familiar to you, others may be new. It's interesting to note that many of the new ingredients have been in use in various cultures for many, many years.

Adzuki beans
Adzuki beans are small and very compact, with a deep reddish-brown color. These tiny beans are a staple in the Far East and revered in Japan for their healing properties. They are low in fat and reputed to be more digestible than most other beans, as well as rich sources of potassium and iron and B vitamins (but not B12).

Agar-agar
Agar-agar flakes are made from a type of sea vegetable. They are nature's alternative to "gelatine" and are used to make delicious fruit kanten.

Amasake
A fermented sweet rice drink with the texture of milk. It is a creamy base for custards, puddings and frostings, not to mention a wonderfully satisfying drink and good source of complex carbohydrates on its own.

Arame
A large leafy sea vegetable, arame is finely shredded and boiled before drying and packed for selling. Since it is precooked, it requires far less cooking time than other sea vegetables and can be marinated for salads with no cooking at all. One of the milder-tasting sea plants, it is a great source of protein and the minerals calcium and potassium.

Avocado oil
Monounsaturated oil made from pressing whole avocados. Perfect for sautéing, frying, baking and other cooking. The mild flavor is perfect for just about any dish and its stability under heat makes it essential cooking oil.

Balsamic vinegar
Italian vinegar made from white trebbiano grapes. Natural balsamic vinegar is rich in live bacteria and enzymes that aid digestion.

Bancha
This Japanese tea made from the stems and twigs of the tea bush has no caffeine and is packed with antioxidants.

Barley
Barley is the oldest cultivated grain and serves to make everything from malted whisky to tea and miso. However, by itself, barley is a great low-fat grain full of nutrients and helps the body in breaking down fat. Delicious when cooked with other whole grains and in soups and salads.

Barley malt
A sweetener or grain honey made from sprouted barley that is cooked into sweet syrup. The syrup contains dextrin, maltose, various minerals and protein.

Black soybeans
Rounder and plumper than other varieties, black soybeans are renowned in Asia for their restorative effects on the reproductive organs. Incredibly sweet and rich, but requiring roasting and a long cooking time.

Bran
A fiber-rich layer just beneath the hull of whole grains that protects the endosperm or germ. Bran is a good source of calcium, carbohydrates and phosphorous and is the main reason for eating grains in their whole form.

Brown rice (see rice)

Buckwheat (kasha)
A very strengthening and warming grain containing more protein than most other grains, as well as iron and B vitamins. Buckwheat is good for high blood pressure and other circulatory difficulties.

Bulgur (cracked wheat)
Bulgar is made from wholewheat berries that are cracked into pieces, which enables it to cook quite quickly. It is a great breakfast cereal in place of porridge for a pleasant change. Bulgur is most commonly associated with tubule, a marinated grain salad combining tomatoes, onions, cucumbers and olive oil dressing.

Burdock
A wild, hearty plant from the thistle family. This long dark-brown root is renowned as one of nature's finest blood purifiers and skin clarifiers. A strong, dense root vegetable, burdock has a very centering, grounding energy and is most commonly used in stews and long-simmered sautés.

Cannellini beans
Creamy white oval beans most commonly used in the Italian dish *pasta e fagiol*. Their creamy texture makes them ideal for purées, dips and creamy soups.

Chestnuts
The rich texture and taste of chestnuts belie the fact that they are low in fat, making them an ideal ingredient in many recipes. At their peak in the autumn, fresh chestnuts are a wonderful addition to soups, stews and vegetable dishes, and their natural sweet taste makes them a great dessert ingredient. As a complex carbohydrate they release energy slowly into the bloodstream.

Chickpeas (garbanzo beans)
Chickpeas have a rich texture and creamy taste when cooked, and taste wonderful when used for making hummus – a creamy spread, combining chickpeas, olive oil, tahini, lemon juice and a bit of garlic. Also fantastic for including in bean dishes, combined with sweet vegetables or corn, as well as in soups and stews.

Daikon
A long white radish root with a peppery taste. Used in soups, salads and stews, and an ingredient of medicinal drinks. It is reputed to aid in the digestion of fat and protein, as well as helping the body assimilate oil and cleanse organ tissue. Also available in a dried shredded form.

Dashi stock
Dashi stock is an essential ingredient in macrobiotic dishes and Japanese cuisine. It is an earthy-flavored stock made from kombu soaking water, and a great base for soups, stews, sauces, noodle broths and dips. Usually dashi is seasoned to taste with a generous serving of shoyu. Often mirin is also added, plus a little juice squeezed from a piece of grated ginger root. This simple soup stock can be stored in the refrigerator and used for several days. With additional vegetables it can be used as a clear broth, served hot or cold.

Dulse
Dried dulse is another great sea vegetable for adding depth of flavor to soups, stews, salads and bean stews. It has a rich red color and is high in potassium.

EFAs (essential fatty acids)
These include omega-3, omega-6 and omega-9 fatty acids and are the "good" fats that we must obtain from our diet. Omega-6 and omega-9 are found in most foods, but omega-3 is somewhat elusive and only found in certain nuts, seeds and cold-water fish.

Flaxseeds
Rich in vitamin E and richer than soybeans in omega-3 fatty acids, flaxseeds have a sweet, nutty flavor. On their own, flaxseeds can have a laxative effect on the body. Many vegans enjoy them daily for the omega-3 benefits.

Fu
A meat substitute developed by vegetarian Buddhist monks, Fu is made of dried wheat gluten. It is a good low-fat source of protein and can be used in various soups and stews by simply reconstituting it with added water.

Ginger
A spicy golden-colored root vegetable with a variety of uses in cooking. It imparts a mild, peppery taste to cooking and is commonly used in stir-fries, sautés, sauces and dressings. Shaped like fingers of a hand, ginger has the reputation of stimulating circulation with its hot taste. A very popular remedy in Oriental medicine for helping with everything from joint pain to stomachache and acid indigestion.

Gluten
The protein found in wheat, although it is also found in smaller amounts in other grains such as barley, oats and rye. When kneaded in dough, gluten becomes elastic and holds air pockets that are released by the leavening, helping the bread to rise. Gluten is also used to prepare seitan, a meat substitute made from wheat gluten.

Hijiki
Sold in its dry form, hijiki resembles black angel-hair pasta. It is one of the strongest tasting of all sea plants, but soaking it for several minutes before cooking can tame its briny flavor. Hijiki is one of the richest sources of useable calcium in the plant kingdom, with a huge amount of calcium per half cup. It has no saturated fat and is great for weight-loss programs.

Kombu

A sea vegetable packaged in wide, dark, dehydrated strips that will double in size when soaked and cooked. Kombu is a great source of glutamic acid – a natural flavor enhancer – so adding a small piece to soups and stews deepens flavors. It is also generally believed that kombu improves the digestibility of grains and beans when added to these foods in small amounts.

Kuzu

A high-quality starch made from the root of the kuzu plant, native to the mountains of Japan. Kuzu grows like a vine with tough roots. Used primarily as a thickener, this strong root is reputed to strengthen the digestive tract due to its alkaline nature.

Legumes

A large plant family including beans, lentils, peanuts and peas.

Lentils

An ancient legume that comes in many varieties, such as common brown-green, red, yellow and French green, or puy (a tiny sweet variety, which is also great in salads). Very high in protein and minerals and having a full-bodied peppery taste, lentils are enjoyable in everything from stews and soups to salads and side dishes.

Maitake mushrooms

Maitake are considered to be the king of mushrooms, because they are so delicious and have a reputation as a very powerful healing food. Enjoy them in soups, stews and teas. Medical researchers have been studying the anti-tumor activity of these mushrooms for many years. Simply put, they can activate the immune system's T-cells, which travel the bloodstream seeking and destroying cancer cells.

Millet

Millet is a tiny grain native to Asia. An effective alkalizing agent, it is the only whole grain that does not produce stomach acids, so it aids spleen and pancreas function as well as stomach upset. Millet is very versatile, used for making delicious grain dishes, creamy soups, stews and porridges. With its sweet nutty taste and beautiful yellow color, it complements most foods but goes best with sweet vegetables such as squash and corn.

Mirin

Japanese rice wine with a sweet taste and very low alcohol content. Made by fermenting sweet brown rice with water and koji (a cultured rice), mirin adds depth and dimension to sauces, glazes and various other dishes, and can be used as a substitute for sherry in cooking.

Miso

A fermented soybean paste used traditionally to flavor soups but prized throughout Asia for its ability to strengthen the digestive system. Traditionally aged miso is a great source of high-quality protein. Miso is available in a wide variety of flavors and strengths, but the most nutritious kind is made from barley and soybeans and aged for at least two years. Miso is rich in digestive enzymes that are delicate and should not be boiled. Just lightly simmering miso activates and releases the enzymes, releasing its strengthening qualities into food.

Miso bouillon
A ready-made stock which adds richness to soups and stews. It is available in natural food stores. If not available, use a natural vegetable bouillon stock cube.

Mochi
Mochi is made by cooking sweet brown rice and then pounding or extruding it to break the grains, a process that results in a very sticky substance. Mochi can be used to make creamy sauces or to give the effect of melted cheese, or simply cut into small squares and pan fried, creating tiny turnover-like puffs, which are a rich source of complex carbohydrates. Delicious when dipped into malt barley syrup or rice syrup.

Mung beans
Tiny pea-shaped deep-green beans, mung are most popular in their sprouted forms, although they cook up quickly, making delightful soups and purées. Mung bean sprouts are a delicious addition to any salad or stir-fried dish.

Nori (sea laver)
Usually sold in paper-thin sheets, nori is a great source of protein and minerals such as calcium and iron. Most well known as a principal ingredient of sushi, nori has a mild, sweet flavor, just slightly reminiscent of the ocean. Great for strengthening grain and noodle dishes, floating in soup or adding to stir-fries.

Nut butters
Thick pastes made from ground nuts. While rich in fiber and protein, nut butters are also excellent sources of good-quality fat. Nut butters have intense, rich flavors and are great in sauces, dressings and baked goods.

Nuts
Nuts are true powerhouses of energy. Bearing in mind that, in most cases, nuts have the strength to grow entire trees, imagine what impact they have on us, giving us great strength and vitality. In small amounts (being calorifically dense), they are wonderful for taste and richness, and for a lift of energy.

Oats
Containing high amounts of protein and rich in B vitamins, oats are good to use in soups in the winter or for morning porridge.

Oil
Oils are rich liquids extracted from nuts, seeds, grains and fruit (such as olives and avocados). A highly refined food source, oils add a rich taste to foods, making dishes more satisfying and creating a warming, vitalizing energy and soft supple skin and hair. Try to choose oils that are cold pressed since these oils have been extracted by pressing and not by extreme heat, which can render oil carcinogenic.

Quinoa
A tiny seed-like grain native to the Andes Mountains, pronounced keen-wah, this small grain packs in it a powerhouse of protein and numerous amino acids not normally found in large amounts in most whole grains, particularly the amino acid lysine, which aids digestion. Quinoa grains are quite delicate, so nature has coated them with an oily substance called *saponin*. If the grain isn't rinsed well, it can have a bitter taste. Quinoa has a lovely nutty taste and cooks quickly, qualities that make it a great wholegrain addition to your menus.

Rice
The staple grain of many cultures, rice is low in fat and rich in vitamins, amino acids and minerals, containing calcium, protein, iron, and B vitamins. Rice as we know it was reportedly cultivated in India and spread from there to Asia and the Middle East. In its whole form, rice is a near-perfect food. High in moisture, rice acts like a gentle diuretic, balancing the moisture content of the body and encouraging the elimination of any excess. There are limitless uses of brown rice as the staple grain in daily cooking. It can be pressure cooked, steamed, boiled, fried, baked, roasted or sautéed, and used in breads, sushi, casseroles, sautés, pilafs or stuffings.

Rice milk
A creamy liquid made by cooking ten parts water to one part rice for 1 hour. The resulting rice is pressed through a cheese-cloth, creating "milk." It is also commercially available.

Rice syrup
Also known as *brown rice syrup, rice malt* or *yinnie*, rice syrup is a thick amber syrup made by combining sprouted barley with cooked brown rice and storing it in a warm place. Fermentation begins and the starches in the rice are converted to maltose and some other complex sugars, making this syrup a wonderfully healthy sweetener. Complex sugars release slowly into the blood stream, providing fuel for the body, rather than wreaking havoc on blood sugar levels. Rice syrup's wonderful, delicate sweetness makes it ideal for baked goods and other desserts. The Japanese call this syrup "liquid sweetness."

Salt
The quality of salt we use is important – the best one is white unrefined sea salt with no additives. Unrefined salts are rich in trace minerals such as magnesium, zinc and selenium, which have been destroyed in processed salt.

Sea vegetables
Exotic vegetables harvested from the sea coast and nearby rocks, high in protein and rich in minerals. Readily available in dehydrated form in natural foods stores, sea vegetables are not yet widely used but are growing in popularity for their nutritional benefits and interesting taste.

Seeds
In a word, seeds are powerhouses. Remember that they are the source of entire plants, even trees in some cases. That's a lot of energy in a little seed. They are good sources of protein and calcium but, because of their high oil content, they spoil relatively quickly and are best kept refrigerated. The most popular seeds in natural foods cooking include pumpkin, poppy, sunflower and sesame.

Seitan (wheat gluten)
Most commonly called *wheat meat*, seitan is made from wheat gluten by kneading the bran and starch out of flour. Raw seitan is rather bland, so most commercial brands are simmered in savory broth before sale. A wonderful source of protein, seitan is low in calories and fat, and very popular in Asian "mock meat" dishes as well as hearty stews and casseroles.

Sesame tahini
A thick, creamy paste made from ground hulled sesame seeds, sesame tahini is used for flavoring everything from sauces and salad dressings to dips, spreads and baked goods.

Shiso (beefsteak leaf)
A lovely herb, rich in calcium and iron, with large reddish leaves. A popular staple in Japan, shiso is often used in pickling, most commonly in umeboshi plum pickling.

Shitake mushrooms
Shitake are loaded with nutrition and very powerful for lowering cholesterol and triglyceride levels and for cleansing blood. Scientists have recently isolated substances from shitake that may play a role in the cure and prevention of heart disease, cancer and AIDS. Shitake mushrooms can be found in natural food stores. They have an intensely earthy taste so a few go a long way. Before cooking, it is necessary to soak the dried ones for about 20 minutes until tender. The soaking water can be used later, but trim off the stems as they can be bitter tasting. Shitake are wonderful in soups, stews, gravies, sauces and medicinal teas.

Shoyu (soy sauce)
A confusing title because it is the generic term for Japanese soy sauce as well as the name of a specific type of traditionally made soy sauce, the distinguishing characteristic of which is the use of cracked wheat as the fermenting starter, along with soybeans. The best shoyu is aged for at least two years. It is high in glutamic acid, a natural form of monosodium glutamate (MSG), which makes it an excellent flavor enhancer and great for marinating, pickling and sautéing. Shoyu is a lighter seasoning than tamari.

Soba
A noodle made from buckwheat flour. Some varieties contain other ingredients, such as wheat flour or yam flour, but the best-quality soba noodles are those made primarily of buckwheat flour.

Soybeans
The base for many natural foods products, from miso, tofu and tempeh to soy sauce, soy milk and soy flour. On their own, soybeans are rather bland and hard to digest, so are more commonly used in other products. However, when cooked on their own (long and slow cooking is the only way), soybeans are most delicious.

Soy foods
A catchall term for the wide range of foods that have soybeans as their base: soy milk, tofu, tempeh, soy sauce, tamari, shoyu, miso, soy cheese, soy oil, and so forth.

Soy milk
Soy milk is sometimes used in baking and making desserts. It is a processed soybean, which can be difficult to digest if used on a regular basis or taken as a drink, but it works well for baking. It is preferable to use rice, oat or almond milk with breakfast cereals.

Soy sauce
Traditional soy sauce (the same as shoyu) is the product of fermenting soybeans, water, salt and wheat. Containing salt and glutamic acid, soy sauce is a natural flavor enhancer. The finest soy sauces are aged from one to two years, like tamari and shoyu, while commercial soy sauce is synthetically aged in a matter of days, producing a salty artificial-flavored condiment.

Tamari
A fermented soy sauce product that is actually the liquid that rises to the top of the keg when making miso. This thick, rich flavor enhancer is nowadays produced by a fermentation process similar to that of shoyu, but the starter is wheat free. Tamari is richer, with a full-bodied taste, and contains more amino acids than regular soy sauce.

Tempeh
A traditional Indonesian soy product, created by fermenting split cooked soybeans with a starter. As the tempeh ferments, a white mycelium of enzymes develops on the surface, making the soybeans more digestible, as well as providing a healthy range of B vitamins. Tempeh can be used for everything from sandwiches and salads to stews and casseroles.

Toasted (dark) sesame oil
This oil, extracted from toasted sesame seeds, imparts a wonderful nutty flavor to quick sautés, stir-fries and sauces, but should not be cooked over a high heat for a long period.

Tofu (soybean curd)
Tofu is a wonderful source of protein and phytoestrogens, and very versatile. Rich in calcium and cholesterol free, tofu is made by extracting the curd from coagulated soy milk and then pressing it into bricks. Tofu can be used in everything from soups and stews to salads, casseroles and quiches, or as the creamy base of sauces and dressings. It absorbs the tastes of other foods that are cooked with it and is especially nice in a marinade.

Udon
Udon are flat noodles, much like fettuccine, and may be entirely wholewheat or come in a variety of blends of flours, including brown rice, lotus root and unbleached white flour. I use the wholewheat variety.

Umeboshi paste
A purée made from umeboshi plums to create a concentrated condiment. Use sparingly as it is quite salty, but it is great for using as an ingredient in salad dressings and sauces, or for spreading on corn on the cob.

Umeboshi plums
Japanese pickles (actually green apricots) with a fruity, salty taste. Pickled in a salt brine and shiso leaves for at least a year (the longer the better), umeboshi (or umi) plums are traditionally served as a condiment with various dishes, including grains. Umeboshi plums are reputed to aid in the healing of a wide array of ailments from stomachaches to migraines, because they alkalize the blood. These little red plums (turned red by the shiso leaves) add vitamin C and iron, and make good preservatives.

Umeboshi vinegar (ume su)
A salty liquid left over from pickling umeboshi plums. Used as vinegar, it is great for salad dressings and pickling.

Vinegar (brown rice)
A fermented condiment. Although lots of vinegars exist, they can be very acidic. I use brown rice vinegar made from fermented brown rice and sweet brown rice, umeboshi vinegar and balsamic vinegar. Great for reducing lactic acid in the body.

Wakame
A very delicate member of the kelp family, wakame is most traditionally used in miso soups and salads. It requires only a brief soaking and short cooking time. With a gentle flavor, wakame is a great way to introduce sea vegetables to your diet.

Wheat
Called the "staff of life," wheat has been the mainstay of foods in temperate climates since the dawn of time. There are many strains of wheat, classified according to hardness or softness, which reflects the percentage of protein content. Hard winter wheat is high in gluten and is best for breads, while softer wheat works best in pastries.

Wholewheat flour
A flour ground from wholewheat berries that is high in gluten. Good stoneground flour retains much of its germ and bran, and therefore much more of its nutrients, than its unbleached white counterpart, making it a healthier choice.

Zest
Also called peel, zest is the thin colored layer of skin on citrus fruit that imparts a fragrant essence of the fruit into whatever is being cooked.

BIBLIOGRAPHY

American Institute for Cancer Research/World Cancer Research Fund 2009–11. "Nutritional and lifestyle characteristics of vegetarian and very low meat diets as determinants of subsequent cancer risk."

Bingham, S. et al. 2007. "Epidemiologic assessment of sugars consumption using biomarkers: Comparisons of obese and nonobese individuals in the European Prospective Investigation of Cancer Norfolk," *Cancer Epidemiol Biomarkers Prev* 16(8).

Brown, S. 2009. *Modern Day Macrobiotics*. North Atlantic Books.

Campbell, T.C. & Campbell, T.M. 2006. *The China Study*. BenBella Books.

Castelli, W. 2011. *Framingham Heart Study*. http://www.framinghamheartstudy.org.

Cho, E. et al. 2003. "Premenopausal fat intake and risk of breast cancer," *Journal of the National Cancer Institute* 95(14).

DeMaris, S. 2009. *Macro Magic for Kids and Parents*. Cedar Tree Books.

Department of Health 2000. *An Organisation with a Memory*. The Stationery Office (TSO).

Duke, J. 1999. Research for the U.S. Department of Agriculture (USDA), *Journal of Alternative Complementary Medicine*.

Hirayama, T. 1971. "Epidemiology of stomach cancer," in Murakami, T. (ed.), *Early Gastric Cancer* (Gann Monograph on Cancer Research No. 11), pp. 3–19. University of Tokyo Press.

Hirayama, T. 1981. "Relationship of soybean paste soup intake to gastric cancer risk," *Nutrition and Cancer* 3, pp. 223–33.

Ito, A. 1989. "Protection miso offers to those exposed to radiation," research carried out at Hiroshima University's Atomic Radioactivity Medical Laboratory (http://yufoundation.org/furo.pdf).

Kushi, A., Tara, B., Esko, E., Spear, W. & Snyder, M. 1981. "Standard Macrobiotic Diet." Kushi Institute (http://www.kushiinstitute.org).

Kushi, A. & Esko, W. 1989. *The Quick and Natural Macrobiotic Cookbook*. McGraw Hill Books.

Kushi, M. 1983. *Your Face Never Lies*. Avery Books.

Kushi, M. & Jack, A. 2003. *The Macrobiotic Path to Total Health*. Random House Publishing.

Lappé, F.M. 1991. *Diet for a Small Planet* (20th Anniversary Edition). Ballantine Books.

Messina, M. & Barnes, S. 1991. "The role of soy products in reducing risk of cancer," *Journal of the National Cancer Institute* 83, pp. 541–46.

Nishimura, M. 2010. *Mayumi's Kitchen*. Kodansha Publishing.

Pirello, C. 2007. *Cooking the Wholefoods Way*. H.P. Books.

Pirello, C. 2009. *This Crazy Vegan Life*. Penguin Group.

Robbins, J. 1987. *Diet for a New America*. HJ Kramer.

Sacks, E.M., Caste, W.P., Dormer, A. & Kass, E.H. 1975. "Plasma lipids and lipoproteins in vegetarians and controls," *New England Journal of Medicine* 292, pp. 1148–5.

Tara, B. 1982. *Macrobiotics and Human Behavior*. Japan Publications.

Tara, B. 2008. *Natural Body, Natural Mind*. Xlibris Corporation.

Tara, B. 2011. Website: http://www.billtara.net. For current details of our Macrobiotic Health Coaching Programme, please visit my website.

U.N. Food and Agriculture Organization (FAO). 2006. "The state of food insecurity in the world 2006: Eradicating world hunger – taking stock ten years after the World Food Summit." Available at: http://www.fao.org/docrep/009/a0750e/a0750e00.htm.

Varona, V. 2009. *Macrobiotics for Dummies*. Wiley Publishing.

Vincent, C., Neale, G. & Woloshynowych, M. 2001. "Adverse events in British hospitals: Preliminary retrospective review," *British Medical Journal* 322, pp. 517–9.

Watson-Tara, M. 2011. Website: www.marlenewatsontara.com. For details of workshops, programs and seminars, please contact me via my website.

World Cancer Research Fund. 2011. "Food, nutrition, physical activity and the prevention of cancer: A global perspective," *Expert Report*.

World Health Organization. 2002. "The World Health Report 2002: Reducing risks, promoting healthy life." Available at: http://www.who.int/whr/2002/en.

World Health Organization. 2011. "WHO global status report on noncommunicable diseases, 2010." Available at: http://www.who.int/topics/diet/en.

Yamamoto, S. 2002. "Cancer information and epidemiology division," PhD thesis, National Cancer Center Research Institute,Tokyo.

Yamamoto, S. et al. 1974. "Antitumor effect of seaweeds," *Japanese Journal of Experimental Medicine* 44, pp. 543–46.

Yudkin, J. 1972. *Pure, White and Deadly*. Davis-Poynter Ltd.

Zeenews.com. 2010. "Cavemen ground flour, prepared veggies 30,000 years ago." Available at: http://zeenews.india.com/news/from-the-past/cavemen-ground-flour-prepared-veggies-30-000-years-ago_662428.html.

Zhao, X. 2006. *Reflections of the Moon on Water*. Virago Press.

INDEX OF RECIPES

Marlene's Macro Shopping List

This shopping list is something to works towards, so do not be overwhelmed and feel you have to rush off to the shops and buy everything today. It is, however, a good idea to start replacing items from your kitchen cupboard with all these new delicious healthy ingredients below.

Take a look inside Marlene's kitchen ...

Agar-Agar
Almond Extract, Vanilla Extract
Adzuki Beans
Balsamic Vinegar
Bancha Twig Tea
Barley
Barley Malt Syrup
Brown Rice Miso or Barley Miso
Brown Rice Syrup
Brown Rice Vinegar
Bulgur
Chickpeas, Organic, Dried or Canned
Couscous
Dried Burdock Root
Dried Daikon
Dried Fruit (Raisins and Prunes)
Dried Lotus Root
Dried Maitake Mushrooms
Dried Shitake Mushrooms
Extra Virgin Olive Oil
Green Lentils
Hazelnut Butter
Kidney Beans, Organic, Dried or Canned
Kuzu
Millet
Organic Peanut Butter
Organic Soy Sauce, such as Shoyu or Tamari
Organic Sunflower Oil for Deep Frying
Tempura
Quinoa
Red Lentils
Rice Mirin
Seitan
Selection of Dried Herbs
Sesame Oil
Short-Grain Brown Rice
Soba Noodles
Sweet White Miso
Tahini
Tempeh
Toasted Dark Sesame Oil
Tofu

Udon Noodles
Umeboshi Paste
Umeboshi Plum
Umeboshi Vinegar
Unrefined Sea Salt

Sea Vegetables
Arame
Dulse
Hijiki
Kombu
Nori
Wakame

Nuts and Seeds
Almonds
Chia Seeds
Pumpkin
Sesame
Walnuts

Vegetables and Fruit I Use, Varying Them Most Days for Soups, Stews and Stir-Fries
Apples
Artichokes (In Season)
Arugula
Basil (In Season)
Berries (In Season)
Broccoli
Cabbage
Carrots
Celery
Chard
Cucumber
Fennel
Fresh Ginger
Fresh Corn (In Season)
Garlic
Kale
Leeks
Lemons
Lettuce
Onions
Oranges
Parsley
Pears
Radishes
Romanesco Broccoli
Sauerkraut
Scallions
Squash or Pumpkin
Watercress

Macrobiotic Health Coach Training

People are waking up to the need for healthy living and this calls for someone to guide them through the fads and confusion. Are you up to the challenge?

The dramatic rise in degenerative disease attributed to diet and lifestyle has created a demand for ways of addressing disease prevention and personal health maintenance. Health coaching is a specific process which helps clients to identify health goals and offers support in achieving them, in part by providing a practical plan of self-generated action. Our Health Coach intensive course will prepare you to carry out this mission.

Our course embodies the most up-to-date principles of macrobiotic health care and represents a unique blend of ancient wisdom and modern insight. As well as practitioner training, students will receive training in:

✿   Macrobiotic nutrition for health and recovery

✿   The principles of human ecology

✿   Oriental diagnosis and health assessment

✿   Natural foods cooking and home remedies

✿   Basic shiatsu massage

✿   Body energy and movement

The complete course comprises over 100 hours of classroom instruction and includes a full complement of workbooks and assignments for home study. Our teachers are experts in their field and can draw on a minimum of thirty years' personal experience in their particular areas of expertise.

Teachers of cooking, yoga and personal development, or anyone in the helping professions, can use these skills to add value and an extra dimension to their practice. The course will also serve dedicated individuals who simply want to increase their knowledge of health for themselves and their family. Would you like to learn how?

For dates and prices of our next Macrobiotic Health Coach Training program, contact us at **marlenewt@hotmail.co.uk or ww.tara@msn.com**

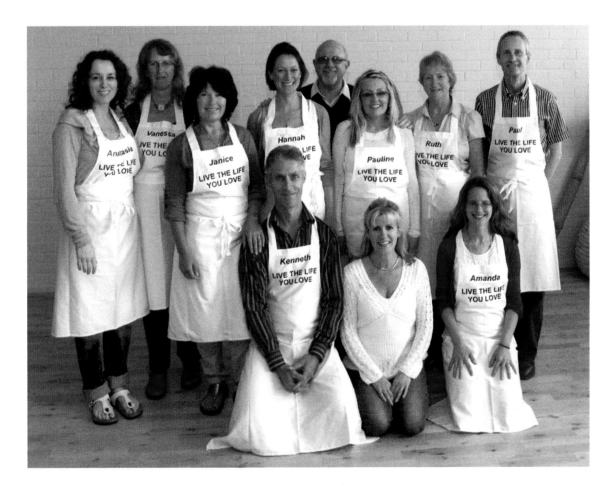

Our graduates from the class of 2011 Macrobiotic Health Coaching Program.

Student comments:

"You've got it all with Bill and Marlene: mind, body and spirit. The first steps towards the great life to which we all aspire." **Kenneth, Paris**

"Bill and Marlene share their wealth of knowledge in a way that I too want to share all that I have learnt from them on the macrobiotic coaching course. As a shiatsu practitioner, I now can motivate others who want to help themselves move away from old habits of eating into new habits that will then enhance their life." **Vanessa, Scotland**

"This is a truly powerful and transformational course led by Bill and Marlene, who are world-class practitioners. I am feeling ever more ready to support others to achieve their own optimum health and well-being. I challenge anyone to leave this course unchanged for the better!" **Amanda, Helensburgh, Scotland**

Macrobiotic Health Services

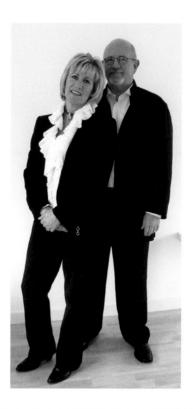

BILL TARA & MARLENE WATSON-TARA

✿ Individual Health Consultations

✿ Women's Health Programs

✿ Weight Loss Circle

✿ Lectures & Workshops

✿ Cooking Classes

Bill and Marlene are international teachers of natural approaches to health and healing. Between them they represent over seventy years of experience and research working with both individuals and large groups.

If you would like to maintain the highest degree of health for you and your family or are dealing with chronic health issues, they can help you design a program that fits your unique needs.

Visit Marlene's website, www.marlenewatsontara.com, or Bill at www.billtara.net.